Brief Psychotherapy with the Latino Immigrant Client

New, Recent, and Forthcoming Titles
of Related Interest

Brief Psychotherapy with the Latino Immigrant Client

Marlene D. de Rios, PhD

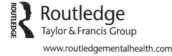

Routledge
Taylor & Francis Group
www.routledgementalhealth.com

The Haworth Press, Inc., 10 Alice Street, Binghamton, NY 13904–1580

Cover design by Marylouise E. Doyle.

Library of Congress Cataloging-in-Publication Data

Dobkin de Rios, Marlene.
  Brief psychotherapy with the Latino immigrant client / Marlene D. de Rios.
    p. cm.
  Includes bibliographical references and index.
  ISBN 0-7890-1089-5 (hard : alk. paper) — ISBN 0-7890-1090-9 (soft . alk. paper)
    1. Hispanic Americans—Mental health services. 2. Brief psychotherapy. 3. Immigrants—Mental health services—United States. 4. Hispanic Americans—Mental health. I. Title.

RC451.5.H57 D63 2000
616.89'14'08968073—dc21

                                                                          00-033531

CONTENTS

ABOUT THE AUTHOR

Marlene D. de Rios, PhD, is Professor Emerita at California State University at Fullerton, where she has taught medical and psychological anthropology and cross-cultural psychopathology. She is also Associate Clinical Professor in the Department of Psychiatry & Human Behavior at the University of California at Irvine, teaching transcultural psychiatry and hypnosis.

Dr. de Rios has served as Health Science Administrator at the National Institute of Mental Health in Rockville, Maryland, and as Director of Counseling Services at the Burn Center at the University of California at Irvine's Medical Center. She is a licensed marriage and family counselor in private practice in both Fullerton and Santa Ana, California.

Dr. de Rios is the author of three books and over 200 scientific papers that have been published in books and journals focused on transcultural psychiatry, psychology, medical anthropology, botany, and surgery.

Chapter 1

An Anthropologist Becomes a Psychotherapist: Lessons from Shamanistic Healing

The morning dawned with a rooster's crow. It was 1978. I heard my father-in-law, Don Hilde, get up (it was 6:00 a.m.), as a knock sounded on the clinic door in his ramshackle house located in the outskirts of the small Amazonian city of Pucallpa, Peru. It signaled the entry of his first patient of the day. As a medical anthropologist and the wife of his oldest son, Yando, whom I met when I studied healing in Iquitos, Peru, some ten years earlier, I watched from early in the morning to late at night as this traditional third world urban folk healer treated men, women, and children tormented by physical and psychological disorders. His clients' problems ran the entire gamut of a psychiatric manual, from marital troubles, to psychotic behaviors, to drug and alcohol abuse, to depression and anxiety. He even treated witchcraft hexes and rectified his clients' misfortunes. To ensure success in my research, I acted as an intake nurse might in a hospital clinic and busily gathered data for my sabbatical research project by administering a questionnaire to all Don Hilde's patients—almost 100 people—for a month, as they sought help from this urban shaman. I discovered a new culture-specific disorder, called *saladera,* which I wrote about for a cultural psychiatry journal.

Over the years, as I continued my studies of folk healing, called in Spanish *curanderismo,* and traditional Peruvian folk healing, and as I taught university courses on medical anthropology and traditional healing, I never imagined that I would return to graduate school and become a psychotherapist myself. As time went on, however, I felt impelled to see if I could use the knowledge that I had gained living among traditional shamanic healers, in third world Amazonian slums, in a practical hands-on way in my own society. Nor did I realize in the 1980s when I began my second career as a psychotherapist that my field experiences in the Amazon and on the coast of Peru where I studied with more than twenty-five different traditional healers would provide me with a set of strategies to help me as I began to treat Latino immigrants in Southern California.

This manual is the result of the confluence of my two careers—in medical anthropology and clinical psychology. For me, it has been very useful to understand the psychological outlook and stressors facing individuals who were raised in Latin America, and then apply this knowledge to design short-term psychological treatments for recent immigrants now in U.S. urban centers. I hope that this knowledge will serve other therapists as well, Latino or otherwise, who treat the urban immigrant poor—those men and women who escape poverty, a lack of education, and few opportunities for betterment by translocating to a new country. They climb fences, swim rivers, board planes, and somehow manage to set up themselves up in a new environment.

As a Southern California psychotherapist who has worked both in private practice and as part of a multidisciplinary university independent provider association largely involved in time-limited treatment, I have treated Spanish-speaking men, women, and children for the past fifteen years. During the course of working with these clients for three, five, six, or ten visits, I have drawn on my understanding of the third world urban poor to guide me in the assessment and treatment of Latinos, and in particular to develop and use culturally resonant techniques that are meaningful to this population. I lived among similar peoples and experienced and learned about their poverty, their beliefs and values, and the way that their societies were structured, as well as their goals and their hopes for the future. Over the past nine years, licensed as a marriage and family therapist in California, I have treated more than 370 Spanish-speaking individuals, families, and children, most of them referred by managed care organizations. This database forms an ethnographic foundation upon which I offer advice for other psychotherapists to assess and intervene with Latino immigrant clients.

Managed care, with its inherently lower costs to the consumer, has been very popular with growing segments of the Spanish-speaking immigrant community. Access issues regarding this underserved population have changed since Karno and Edgeston's (1969) pioneering studies. Among the working poor, it is becoming more common for at least one member of the family to obtain mental health insurance. Studies of a large national sample of legal immigrants since the Immigration Reform and Control Act of 1986 (IRCA) document that almost 50 percent of such immigrants do have access to health insurance. More and more individuals are finding their way into managed care settings. With or without interpreters, clinicians find that they must acquire new techniques to be successful with these patients.

The majority of my clients have hailed from Mexico, and South and Central America. Puerto Rican and Cuban clients are much fewer in number in the western United States. However, Mexican immigrants constitute more than 80 percent of Latin Americans in the United States, and their numbers greatly impact managed care. I include research findings that heighten diversity issues to distinguish particular needs of all three major Latino groups in the United States: Central and South Americans, Cubans, and Puerto Ricans.

In a seminal article, Dr. Lillian Comas-Diaz (1992) looked at the future of psychotherapy over the next twenty years or so. As with other scholars responding to the "browning of America," she argues that changing demographics in the United States and throughout the world make it essential for us to reform health care delivery so that psychotherapy is resonant and meaningful to the client's cultural background.

Latinos, the fastest growing minority group in the United States, need culturally specific therapies that make sense to them, and which consider their unique sociocultural reality and worldview. Much can be learned from the Latin American tradition of shamanistic healing, which is a time-limited intervention that can assist managed care practitioners. Additionally, we need to carefully assess what techniques will be helpful for this population's mental health treatment.

MEDICAL ANTHROPOLOGY CONCEPTS

Medical anthropologists study the multiple ways that people define and treat mental and physical disorders: from tribal healers in tropical rain forests of Peru, to an Andean highland *curandero* scattering flower petals on the path to capture the lost soul of his client, to the urban healer's fortunetelling diagnosis of the client's distress, to the herbalist's preparation of plant teas for a client, to the spiritist maestro's elaborate curing ritual, to the urban clinic of a large anonymous hospital—there are certain paradigms and beliefs that we can learn about and integrate into our own practice of psychotherapy to make it meaningful to a changing client base. Our choices are few: if we insist upon simply translating old wine into new bottles, our clients will not return or will hesitate to seek help for their psychological distresses and dysfunctions. So many immigrants have pulled up roots and disrupted their lives to start anew elsewhere. They have more than their share of adjustments and accommodations to make to their new environments.

In the new field of clinically applied medical anthropology, mental health providers are drawing on the lessons of anthropology to realize that the cultural background of clients has an important influence on their beliefs, behaviors, perceptions, emotions, family structure, and body image, to name a few. Moreover, no culture is ever homogeneous in a psychological sense, even small-scale tribal societies. The medical anthropologist has to bridge the gap between the biomedical concept of disease—the Western physician's perspective on illness drawn from rational scientific medicine—and patients' perspectives on illness—that is, how their lives have been disrupted, their understandings of their problems, and their expectations of treatment.

Arthur Kleinman (1980), a psychiatrist and medical anthropologist, argues for the importance of understanding clients' explanatory models of their illness and their own concepts of etiology, the timing of the illness, and appropriate treatments. The use of metaphor is a major way that the mental health provider can bridge the realm of his or her own explanatory model of science and biomedicine to the different explanatory world of the client. The mental health provider must have a coherent system of explanation and must find solutions to the client's personal human problems. Any healer's system must symbolically connect to the client's world of personal experience, social relations, and cultural meanings. As Helman (1994) has argued, the healer must activate a symbolic bridge to convince the client that the problem can be explained in terms of the healer's theory. As the sayings *(dichos)* and metaphors in this book will show, we can link the phenomenological world of the Latino immigrant with the symbols and metaphors available to us to relate to the particular problem and situation of the client in treatment. Just as a traditional healer guides therapeutic change by manipulating the symbols of the client's world, the psychotherapist must help the client reevaluate and reframe his or her past and present experiences. This new narrative has been examined by recent therapists who see this new story of their suffering and distress reframed into a success story. The therapist has to set the stage and create a mood of expectation and hope.

What are some of the lessons of shamanistic healing that psychotherapists can incorporate into their assessments and treatments of Latin American immigrants? To answer this question, I turn to my research in traditional shamanistic folk healing in Peru, which I conducted over several periods of fieldwork, in the summer of 1967, from June 1968 to July 1969, during the fall of 1977, and from 1978 to 1979. I also draw upon my university teaching experience in the areas of shamanism and medical anthropology, which I have taught at both the graduate and undergraduate levels. Additionally, I co-edited and contributed to a publication in 1989 on shamanism and altered states of consciousness (de Rios and Winkelman, 1989).

THE BIOLOGY OF HOPE

In my book *Amazon Healer* (de Rios, 1992), which is based on the life and work of one urban healer, Don Hilde (who happens to be my father-in-law), I wrote about folk healers around the world who are involved in health care delivery in third world nations, including Latin America. Indeed, many of the Latino immigrants whom we see in managed care are familiar with their own nation's local traditions of health care—either directly or indirectly. Traditional healing is important because it throws light on a particular culture or cultures and allows us to understand health care systems in different parts of the world. We can understand universal as well as culturally particular features of the healing process as we compare indigenous healing with biomedical and psychiatric care.

Briefly, I want to compare one folk healer, Don Hilde, and his symbolic world with the clients I see in my Southern California private practice. Healers such as Don Hilde are appreciated by their communities for their abilities and skills as counselors, for their knowledge of plant medicines, and for their supposed access to spiritual realms. Many more women than men consult folk healers. Stressors from poverty, unemployment, malnutrition, and overcrowding in the Amazon echo similar stressors in urban America—cities such as Santa Ana or Anaheim, California—which propel clients to seek help. The patients of urban folk healers average two or three visits, not unlike the statistics for the Latino immigrant managed care patients whom I see, who are not psychologically savvy and do not expect long-term treatments. They expect to resolve their problems as quickly as possible. Transference concepts are not easy to document in short-term managed care of Latino immigrants. Recognizing and applying psychoanalytic constructs are just not pertinent in cultures with a high illiteracy rate and a lack of understanding of Freudian concepts.

Don Hilde's patients have had access to cosmopolitan medicine as it is practiced in small cities of the Amazon or even the capital city of Lima. Many of the managed care clients whom I treat have access, as well, to family physicians and specialists as their needs demand. What are the typical procedures that a shamanistic healer such as Don Hilde uses compared to the techniques of psychotherapy? Can we, as psychotherapists, learn from shamans to enhance our own proficiency in treating this population?

For starters, most urban folk healers do not splurge on fancy consultation rooms or display signs of success. Don Hilde's consultation room can only be called a cubbyhole! Perhaps this comes from Latin American concepts of envy *(envidia)* or limited good, meaning that one person's good luck and affluence is often seen as the result of depriving someone else of good fortune. In the summer of 1967, I lived in a Peruvian coastal community, Salas, which was reputed to have more than 100 men and women healers. At that time, I interviewed ten healers, most of whom lived in very modest circumstances. They preferred not to display any wealth, and they meticulously avoided provoking the envy of others who might be motivated to pay a witch to hex them in turn. The only "conspicuous consumption" that I observed was a brick chapel that healers erected to honor St. Cipriano, a presumed Roman Catholic patron saint of folk healers.

Like their shamanic forebears in the rain forest, urban healers such as Don Hilde do not question patients about their symptoms but rather present themselves in an omnipotent, all-knowing manner. Folk healers around the world often enter into trance states, but less frequently in agriculture-based societies. Indeed, among shamanistic healers in rural, agricultural settings, these altered states are quite incidental, except when hallucinogenic plants are used, as in Peru, or in some Brazilian spiritualist religions such as the União do Vegetal. Healers in mestizo cultures of Latin America generally do not engage in trances. Rather they learn spells, formulas, rituals, and techniques to foretell the future, and they use a range of other treatment modalities to heal. Don Hilde and others like him are generally of above-average economic status and may survive more comfortably than the farmers around them who lack a skill that can be converted to cash or that enables them to receive gifts (Winkelman, 1989).

Healers adopt a positive and confident manner, which is expected and even demanded of them. They are renowned for the preparation of medicinal brews, which they give to clients to treat their varied ailments. Don Hilde is no exception. In his backyard he grows therapeutic plants, which he brews each day as his clients patiently wait in his front room. At least once or twice a month, he makes a trip to nearby lagoons where he gathers medicinal plants for further preparation. Teas, poultices, and salves are all commonly provided as part of his overall treatment. Many are mixed with pharmaceutical medicines that he purchases from the numerous stores in his small city's downtown area. The shaman creates rapport with clients in Latin America by providing medications and commanding their trust and respect. The Western psychotherapist, in contrast, needs to show an interest in the effects on clients of drugs being provided by the psychiatrist. It is important, too, to inquire into any additional herbal teas or preparations that the Latino client may be currently taking.

Indeed, a growing area of research interest in pharmaceutical anthropology impacts the Latino immigrant in the United States.

Over the past twenty-five to thirty years, pharmacies have become as common in small Latin American cities as gas stations are in the urban American landscape. International biomedical preparations originating in the United States, Europe, and Asia, available in glossy and colorful packaging, can be purchased without prescription in these pharmacies and are often misused, as no instructions are available for the client to consult.

The presentation of self is an important factor in the success of healers, who must be at ease and have faith in their own abilities. Most healers also have a good network of referrals that they use when their clients need surgery or hospitalization. Don Hilde touts the ability of these important others whom he will call upon to help his client if needed. Surely the psychotherapist, too, must also maintain a good referral network, particularly in employee assistance program (EAP) sessions, where it is expected that the provider will be familiar with community resources and even be expected to document this on billing forms.

In summarizing the success of a healer such as Don Hilde, who sees approximately 4,000 new patients a year, or 0.4 percent of the population of 120,000 in his home of Pucallpa, Peru, we need to understand the general psychological knowledge that folk healers or urban shamans call upon. They work with a culturally attuned symbolic system shared by their patients. They often focus on a natural versus a supernatural etiology of illness. In my work in the United States, interestingly enough, only the occasional Latino immigrant client continues to adhere to beliefs in hexes and *brujeria* (witchcraft). Healers, however, do generate exceptional emotional states in their clients through the clients' expectations and anticipation; on occasion, healers administer and themselves take plants that cause alterations in their normal waking consciousness—hallucinogenic substances—to diagnose illness. The psychiatrists who medicate our clients also create unusual states of consciousness through the medicines that they prescribe. Healers create a biology of hope to marshal the healing resources of the client's immune system by symbolic means. The psychotherapist perhaps unwittingly does the same. We call this a transducer effect, which converts energy from one form to another. In biomedicine, there appears to be little place for metaphors to explain the principles of healing. Our scientific worldview demands that we examine how healing occurs, what the biological markers are, and what actually goes on (Rossi, 1986). The folk healer, however, may not be interested in the cellular event, as it transforms to affective, cognitive, and social-interactional experience. He or she uses metaphors and symbols and is interested in outcomes but not process.

A focus on metaphors and storytelling is a way to enhance the well-being of the Latino immigrant client. This is an appropriate psychological technique and strategy similar to those used by shamanistic healers in non-Western cultures. Chapter 4 details the types of metaphors that are appropriate to particular psychiatric disorders of Latino clients and how they can be incorporated into psychotherapeutic communication. What we can discern is that the acculturative stresses that Latino immigrants face do impact their immune systems. All societies have psychological and social stresses and problems that face their members. When we examine the immune system of an individual, we are obliged to ask, "How does it respond to disease agents? How do belief systems, reiterated in metaphor, influence the immune competence of a person's body?"

Depression, for example, causes changes in the functioning of brain chemicals, and unavoidable stress—the type that gives rise to feelings of helplessness—may cause the depletion of catecholamines at the same time that corticosteroids are released in the body. These depress the immune system. This transducer mechanism shows that when people go through emotional, social, and environmental stresses that bring about changes in their lives, they may indeed experience somatic dysfunction.

Latino immigrants often experience unusual stress, which can lead them to a sense of helplessness, experienced as depression or despair *(desesperación)*. Neurochemically, this translates into catecholamine depletion and a surplus of corticosteroid secretions in the body. The disease process has affective, psychological, neurochemical, and endocrinologic components. Psychotherapists in our society may believe that their interventions are squarely in the realm of mental health, but their interventions affect areas of the client's physical health as well. The psychotherapist working with the Latino immigrant has to check out the physical components of the client's presenting symptoms routinely, especially in light of the lack of psychological sophistication of such clients and a strong somatization focus.

Psychological interventions both in the United States and in third world settings try to modify the psychosocial status of the patient and help in one way or another with the individual's ability to cope. They also modify the individual's stress response. The psychotherapist needs to communicate positive expectations that he or she will be successful with the client.

Healers such as Don Hilde use a range of imaging techniques to treat their clients, not unlike those currently used in Western psychotherapy (Sheik, 1984). Hypnosis is a good example of one such efficacious approach to treat biobehavioral disorders such as autoimmune diseases, asthma, skin disorders, pain, high blood pressure, etc. Perhaps folk healers such as Don Hilde provoke the manufacture of endorphins in their clients. These are natural opiatelike substances that are implicated in shamanistic healing—to mediate pain and ecstasy. A key element in the success of urban shamans throughout the world is the way in which they integrate mind and body issues. They do not distinguish between the treatment of mental disorders and physical ones. The mind-body dichotomy that we accept as a given in our own society has little importance in traditional cultures. In many third world societies undergoing rapid culture change and industrialization, this separation is irrelevant. Psychosomatic and somatic disorders are the main types of problems that traditional healers are called upon to treat. The psychotherapist who works with Latino immigrants needs to inquire into the client's physical problems, aches and pains, high blood pressure, etc., as a measure of the level of stress that that person is currently experiencing, without fear of going beyond the scope of his or her license. Think of the psychotherapist as a traffic policeman who directs the client to the appropriate professional for his or her psychosomatic dysfunctions, even though the stressors may be psychological in nature. Nor is it unusual for the primary care physician to make the referral for mental health evaluation and treatment when he or she finds no biological markers to explain the patient's somatic symptoms.

Like shamanistic healers, the psychotherapist must be quick to recognize the interdependence of mind and body and see many somatic disorders as the expression of psychological distress. If a person's body is about to break down, it will do so in its most vulnerable area. Behavioral medicine reiterates the importance of focusing on the interdependence of mind and body. Healers such as Don Hilde use imagery to affect cures and link mind and body ailments. Images can arouse very strong emotions. In Amazonian society, witchcraft hexes and bewitchment fears are primary concerns. For the Latino immigrant, the stressors can be quite different and include inadequate housing, unstable or dangerous work conditions, and nutritional issues as well as other unmet acculturation needs.

In the behavioral medical literature, writers discuss helplessness, hopelessness, and loss as important variables that can be linked to clinical depression. Shamanic healers' concept of mind-body integration leads to the effectiveness of their interventions. Healers try to reverse negative feelings in their clients by alleviating the helplessness and hopelessness that the individual experiences, even though "magical" techniques may be used.

The therapeutic alliance in shamanistic healing appears fragile and distant. It is often difficult to find anything that resembles transference in Don Hilde's Amazon clinic, for example, since the healer does not interact much with clients. The urban shaman rarely knows clients' names, nor does he or she obtain a history regarding their backgrounds or even their presenting symptoms. The amount of time that the healer spends with the patient is very limited as well. However, healers are often older and can be viewed as parental figures. Clients expect that some significant event will occur. The shaman is able to elicit maximum cooperation of the client by posturing or bragging. We see this at its best when the healer's past successes are touted and validated in turn by the referral process in traditional folk healing. This happens when the client, 98 percent of the time, is brought to the folk healer's clinic by a "cured" former patient. The healer's bragging gets the client's immediate attention and offers hope in what may appear to be a hopeless situation. In turn, psychotherapists must not hesitate to sing their own praises and indicate their past accomplishments and professional recognition, as this style of interaction is resonant with indigenous healing traditions.

In Chapters 2 and 3, I go into more detail about the appropriate assessments of the managed care Latino immigrant and what types of therapy are effective. I suggest that three major techniques of intervention are the most successful—hypnosis, behavior modification, and cognitive restructuring. In Chapter 4, I look at concepts from cultural psychology and epistemology, that is, how people know things, especially when they have little education. In this area, metaphors, sayings *(dichos),* stories, and narrative can be effective in communicating ways to change as well as techniques for problem solving. They feed into the transducer effect most powerfully. Chapter 5 provides a typical course of therapy with the Latino immigrant managed care patient, to help the therapist pace and plan an intervention in a timely and appropriate manner. Then in Chapter 6, I turn to specific clinical issues most commonly encountered among Spanish-speaking managed care clients and illustrate them with case studies. In Chapter 7, I draw upon earlier research I conducted with Spanish-speaking immigrants who were alcoholics or who suffered from tuberculosis, to inform the psychotherapist how to best understand the particular dynamics of that clinical population. In Chapter 8, I present a case study of one immigrant, Maria, and her marital and family problems. I look at the effects of working with the Latino immigrant on the non-Latino psychotherapist—namely myself. Chapter 9 sets out some goals and techniques for the non-Latino psychotherapist who treats Latino immigrants.

In the two appendixes, Spanish-language resources are presented as well as the names of published tests and scales. My hypnotic induction for relaxation is presented in Spanish and English and is freely available to the mental health provider to help clients relax and control pain.

Chapter 2

Sociocultural and Psychological Assessment of the Latino Immigrant Managed Care Patient

For psychotherapists to be effective in assessing Spanish-speaking clients, they need to have many different kinds of information about clients at their fingertips. This need is quite different when facing an English-speaking adult or child. That my father was born in Russia, that my mother was a homemaker until I was fourteen years old, that my uncle served with distinction in the armed forces, that my daughter played on her high school volleyball team are all incidental to any psychopathology that I, as an American, might be suffering and for which I could be seeking help. However, when treating a Latino immigrant who originates from a society with multiple social class layers, with different linguistic styles of communication, different ethnic influences and backgrounds, and tightly structured class membership as well as a cultural history of over 400 years of oppression, it is important to assess that client differently than one might a member of one's own society.

In this chapter, I look at the variety of socioeconomic backgrounds of the Latin American immigrant. I focus on communication styles among different segments of the immigrant community, and I examine ethnic identity, value orientations, cultural mores, and health beliefs and practices. Generally, managed care companies do not authorize or pay for psychological testing. Behavior that at first blush may appear pathological to the therapist may be attributable to cultural mores and beliefs, and, thus, a knowledge of Latin American culture is in order at the commencement of any assessment of the client.

To begin with, the psychotherapist must project a sense of *simpatía,* a type of interpersonal style that promotes smooth and pleasant social relationships. A person who is *simpático* has the ability to share other people's feelings and behaves with dignity and respect toward others, avoiding interpersonal conflict (Triandis et al., 1984:1363).

ACCULTURATION STRESS

It is very difficult for immigrants to fit into a new society. They must master new social customs and a new language and learn to negotiate a complex bureaucratic system. Many are unaware of important laws. For example, women in particular may be hesitant to leave an abusive marriage because they are unaware of the protection available to them under U.S. law. Mexican women whom I treat are fearful of leaving a physically abusive husband because in Mexico there is a law against abandoning the home *(abandono del hogar).* Many immigrants do not know that they place themselves in jeopardy if they spank their children the way they might have been spanked themselves when they were young.

In terms of overall immigration statistics, Mexican-born immigrants have the lowest educational attainment of all immigrants from the thirty-eight different countries of origin that the U.S. Department of Commerce reports upon. Only one in four Mexican immigrants has a high school diploma, compared to seven out of ten European or five out of ten African immigrants. Estimates are that between 200,000 and 300,000 immigrants from Mexico alone arrive in the United States each year (Smart and Smart, 1995).

As attempts are made to integrate Latino immigrants into mainstream American life, demands for counseling services will continue to be heavy. The counselor will play a major role in helping Latinos cope with the acculturation stress imposed by their move to the United States. As Quintana (1995) argues, acculturation is not a simple process and is certainly not unidimensional. Berry (1993) has outlined four prototypical acculturation orientations for ethnic minority groups, including integration, assimilation, separation, and marginalization. The ethnic majority groups may themselves value multicultural modes such as assimilation, e.g., the so-called melting pot model, or segregation, as in U.S. history, or even ethnocide, the widespread use of "ethnic cleansing," for example, in the former Yugoslavia. The counselor must assess the Latino immigrant's acculturation orientation early on as well as the predominant orientation of the social, educational, employment, and legal community in which the immigrant lives. Immigrants who have adopted or been forced to adopt separation strategies may need to be referred to an ethnically similar counselor, while immigrants with an assimilation orientation may prefer an American counselor.

Many Latino clients come from rural and relatively isolated areas of the third world and lack urban skills necessary for successful early adaptation. I estimate that about 15 percent of the clients I have seen over the past ten years come from small ranches and isolated villages, away from the mainstream. These individuals have different expectations of therapists than their educated urban counterparts. The less educated person arrives with little or no prior understanding of psychotherapy and its process. Such a person often fails to appear for appointments or at best manages one or two visits with the aim of getting immediate relief for a problem. This person expects the "doctor" to ask questions, to know what is wrong, and to do something. Mainstream medical encounters are often unsatisfying experiences to these clients, as many practitioners do not share or recognize their culture-based expectations. The professionalism of the mainstream health care practitioner may seem cold, impersonal, and uncaring, even hostile. Psychotherapists must see themselves as educators and take that role seriously—in the growing field of acculturation education.

The process of acculturation, as Smart and Smart (1995) argue, is tremendously taxing to the immigrant's ability to cope and adapt. The immigrant has to leave behind a familiar way of life. Latino immigrants differ from their Protestant, northern and western European counterparts in a number of ways. Latino cultures that have a strong mestizo heritage, e.g., Mexico, Peru, Bolivia, Ecuador, and Venezuela, tend to accept and integrate people of varying skin color. The racial discrimination and prejudice that many Latinos face in the

United States is much harsher than anything known in their own cultures.

For example, Roxana learned the hard way what discrimination was. Working as a cook and caretaker for elders in a group home where her lack of English skills was not important, she returned from a group outing and was attacked by gang members in the street. She sustained serious wounds and was rushed to a local hospital, where she was largely ignored and then poorly treated, she thinks, because of her skin color and presumed poverty. Months later, she continued to feel indignant in retelling the incident. I helped her prepare a strongly worded letter of protest to the hospital administrator, and indeed, she received an effusive apology and a promise that the matter would be examined.

These immigrants often lack technical skills to make them competitive in the labor market and there is a heavy reliance on physical labor. This is incongruent with U.S. society, which is fast becoming an information society, not a manufacturing or agricultural one. Immigrants who face acculturation stress find their ability to make decisions with clarity and resolution to be impaired. They also have difficulties in carrying them out effectively. As technology drives greater and greater portions of the U.S. economy, more demanding educational requirements become the norm in hiring American workers. Unskilled Latino immigrants will suffer even more stress in trying to fit in and to meet these higher standards. Moreover, the dominant culture imposes stereotypes and expectations on minority persons—which are insidious forces to keep minorities in their place. Negative stereotypes are pervasive and very much ingrained in the larger society. Members of the dominant society are oblivious to any valid differences between members of minority groups and tend to assign characteristics of the lowest common denominator to all. Immigrants are stigmatized as being less competent. Latinos, faced with this social discrimination, may take a "what's the use" attitude and postpone or abandon plans for study or advancement. People are pushed into barrios that isolate them and mitigate against integration (Smart and Smart, 1995).

SOCIOECONOMIC STATUS
OF THE LATINO CLIENT

As a general rule, it is very important for the psychotherapist to understand the social class background of the patient, whether the client is a rural peasant in a city, an urban laborer at the fringes of modern society in a small town or city in the hinterlands, a savvy wiser-than-his-years urban dweller from a megalopolis such as Mexico City or Guatemala City, the adult child of a Quito businessman, or the son of an Uruguayan diplomat. Individuals in each of the social segments that we can delineate in Latin American society require different treatment and comprehension from the psychotherapist, who must be careful not to stereotype the Latino client simply because he or she possesses few English skills.

Pepe is a good example of a Spanish-speaking immigrant who lives in my area, whose background in philosophy, law, and economics would make the mouth of any of my academic colleagues water. Yet, he works as a school aide, and he and his wife (she also works in the school system) together scrape by with about $25,000 a year. In his home country of Peru, he was a deputy minister of health, he traveled around the country inspecting board and care and resident facilities for indigent poor and retarded individuals, and he had the ear of a minister of Congress. He was enmeshed in a complex network of social relations. Yet, if we were to place him in some kind of socio-economic grid by plotting his income and resident zip code, we might have different expectations about his level of understanding, his psychological knowledge, etc.

Rule #1: Know Thy Patient

Some years ago, the Southern California Association of Governments (1984) did a study of the Los Angeles basin. They predicted that by the year 2000, Latinos would represent 36 percent of the population in the region. By the year 2010, the numbers are expected to rise to 46 percent of the population, with whites in a decided minority. Other studies (National Center for Health Statistics, 1987) have suggested that perhaps as many as 4 million new Spanish-speaking immigrants would come to the Los Angeles area legally before the new millennium as the result of petitions from their relatives who were granted amnesty in 1986. At least eighteen other urban regions of the United States find themselves in similar circumstances, and there are major groupings of Spanish-speaking immigrants in cities throughout the United States, including Miami, New York, Houston, Chicago, Seattle, etc. From the 1960s to the mid-1980s, many writers documented the underuse of social, medical, and psychiatric services by immigrant populations, as well as a high degree of noncompliance with medical advice and interventions. Over the past five years or so, I have been amazed at the speed at which the Spanish-speaking working poor have gravitated to the realm of managed care, especially when the primary wage earner is able to obtain health and mental health insurance. Family therapy is the entry point for most of the other members of the family group, even if only the primary wage earner has insurance coverage. This is now happening as Medicare clients are being contracted for mental health services by large managed care companies such as PacifiCare Behavioral Health and Value Options.

Michael Winkelman (1993), in an important book, *Ethnic Relations in the U.S.,* has summarized the characteristics of the U.S. Latino population, who are now the second largest minority ethnic group. With a high fertility rate, and with an average of four children per family, current estimates of the number of Latinos in the United States are around 30 million. The vast majority of Latin American immigrants are concentrated in California, New Mexico, New Jersey, Arizona, and Texas and generally have urban residence patterns. In fact, more than 80 percent live in cities, often in ethnic urban ghettos where substandard, dilapidated housing can be more costly to rent than standard housing in more affluent neighborhoods. As many as 26 percent of Latinos in the United States lived in poverty in 1994, compared to 12.8 percent of the total U.S. population. Socioeconomic factors have pervasive effects on the adaptation of Latinos to their environment, creating stress and maladaptive responses. This compounds the general problem of acculturation that Spanish-speaking immigrants face as a people.

Winkelman (1993) points out some of the characteristics of this population, where the extended family with a vast network of relatives is slowly being replaced by the nuclear family. A relatively fixed sexual division of labor still remains, with the wife subordinate to the husband. This causes many problems for working wives in the United

States, who often are placed in a double bind. It is hard to prepare the *guisado* (stew) as quickly and as well after nine hours standing in an assembly line, chauffeuring children to sports activities, etc. A high percentage of female-headed households characterize the population (Ruiz, 1995). It is important to understand the role and position of women in the family, especially the role of female children. Are they seen simply as old-age insurance for the mother or father? If so, are we dealing with the "throw-away child" *(desechable)* who in turn presents clinically with a very low sense of self-esteem?

The psychotherapist also must be aware of the range of heterogeneity encountered in the immigrant population. There are many regional, class, educational, and acculturation variations among the rural and urban Spanish-speaking immigrant populations in the United States. It is impossible to generalize, especially with regard to health beliefs and behavior. However, some quick evaluative questions can be placed on the psychotherapist's intake sheet before he or she even greets the new client. At a glance, this data intake can place the patient in a sociocultural matrix, which helps to specify the type of intervention that the psychotherapist needs to make.

For example, it is a good idea to ask clients to identify their place of birth and where they spent the first ten to twelve years of their lives. This helps to understand any modernizing influences that affected them in their early years. A town in Mexico in a difficult-to-pronounce province or a backwater town in El Salvador off the beaten path, will have relatively few links to the outside world. If the name of the community in question is in a Mayan language such as Tzintinzun, or difficult for even the well-traveled tourist to recognize, the psychotherapist should ask the approximate size of the town in which the client was raised. A fair number of my managed care clients come from *ranchos* or hamlets, which may have only ten families in total and may be two or three hours' walk from a village or town.

The case of Jorge illustrates how important it is to understand the client's point of origin when he comes from a small community. He came to see me because of severe depression and paranoia, which occurred after he was falsely accused of theft in the large urban market where he had worked as a janitor for the previous five years. He ended up winning a large out-of-court settlement for defamation of character and false arrest, but the psychological effects on him were tremendous. He began to fear that he was being followed by private investigators, he slept only a few hours a night with a loaded rifle at his side in his living room, and he was prepared to take on anyone who invaded his home. When I assessed his problems, I recognized that the man was illiterate, that he had never been to school, and that he came from a small rural hamlet with only seven other families. Although he was unable to read or write, he had a strong sense of pride in his honesty. The slander against him was a terrible wound to his sense of personal identity.

As I thought about it, I had difficulties at first in understanding his response as I myself had grown up in a large city. I realized from the fieldwork that I had conducted in Peru how important it was to have a sense of belonging to one's community. Being known by everyone there meant that one had to be very careful *never* to steal or one would be pegged for life as a ne'er-do-well. The impact of such slander on Jorge was much worse than it would be on someone with ties to a place where anonymity was the norm—compared to a lifestyle where one's dignity was important irrespective of economic status.

Latino Kinship

What about the socioeconomic structure of the client's family? In many third world countries, a person's family is his or her only available capital. Relatives are expected to help out their family members economically. This value has been called familialism and conceptualizes the individual's possession of a deep sense of belonging and responsibility toward relatives. Individuals also have a sense of family obligation. They strongly identify with and are attached to their nuclear and extended families, and strong feelings of loyalty, reciprocity, and solidarity exist among members of the same family (Simoni and Perez, 1995). The extended family provides an important support network of interdependence among relatives.

Once in the United States, immigrants' remittances home are the backbone of family survival, especially in rural settings where few jobs may be available, or where war makes life difficult for the ones left behind. A client's current economic stresses may be due, in part, to the money he or she sends home, given the duty to support parents and children. Often, an immigrant may remarry and have to deal with a blended family, which is not as common in Latin America as in the United States.

When a woman marries for a second time, she may seriously consider sending her children to live with her parents. Having a grandparent as primary caretaker is not unusual—in fact, it is much more common among Latin American immigrants than among the Anglo patients whom I have treated. Extended family members are crucial to the survival of the family unit, especially when the mother is obliged to work outside the home. Latino women have an important relationship to their mothers, and the grandmother is a pivotal figure with enormous power and influence. This fact will probably continue to have an active and central role in Latino family life (Comas-Diaz, 1992). The psychotherapist must ask, Who lives together and what are the living arrangements?

Monica was ready to leave her husband, Umberto. He had brought his two brothers, one of whom was married with a child, to live with his family in a two-bedroom house, with one bathroom. Monica was very upset by the acting-out behavior of her nine-year-old boy, who had nowhere to call his own, as the married brother had the second bedroom, and everyone in Monica's family had to make do, in a hit-or-miss fashion. Umberto's loyalty to his family of origin took precedence over the minimal creature comforts of his own wife and children. The stress was such that Monica was desperate and ready to separate from her husband. Latina women in these circumstances carry heavy guilt about not keeping the family together despite heavy stressors such as overcrowding.

Poverty variables, too, must be considered in understanding stressors facing the client. Often a neighborhood may be a really dangerous place, with drive-by shootings or drug dealers in alleys and backyards. Children may have to be kept inside the home and their behavior monitored, or else they may develop friendships with gang members or children their age whose older siblings belong to gangs. The clinician needs to assess this phenomenon during intake.

MIGRATION AND MENTAL HEALTH

The process of migration and acculturation leads to disruption in a person's customary life patterns, which can cause psychological distress or symptoms. Favazza (1980) has examined the effects of immigration on mental disorders. He argues that the deprivation associated with culture change directly undermines the security and stability of the family as a functioning system. It produces interpersonal conflicts and alters patterns by which adults socialize their children.

Cristina is a good example. In the United States since the age of sixteen, she had three children, two from an unhappy marriage with an alcoholic husband who beat her and verbally abused all members of the family. The best job that she was able to find kept her out of the house from midnight to dawn, and her fifteen-year-old daughter and seventeen-year-old son were obliged to provide child care for her four-year-old daughter. No wonder her children were "out of control" and the fifteen-year-old was about to run away from home. The seventeen-year-old boy seemed to be a living incarnation of John Travolta in his role in *Saturday Night Fever,* living only for his dancing and "moves."

Children of immigrants with disrupted family structures, in turn, may experience a lack of coherence in their development (Favazza, 1980) and are tentative in their approach to life. They perceive the outer world as atomized into meaningless units, and their inner worlds can become unstructured and fragmented. Some writers, such as Helman (1994), ask if restless, unstable people immigrate more often in an attempt to solve their personal problems. On the other hand, I can argue that there is a positive element to consider, in that immigrants have had to overcome substantial obstacles to move to the United States. Most probably, people who are distressed would not be able to overcome these obstacles (Short et al., 1994). Often left out of the discussion of immigrant mental health, too, is the frame of reference of the hard life left behind in Mexico or elsewhere.

Special life experiences such as war trauma, political oppression, particularly unpleasant migratory experiences, or torture may also provoke mental disorders. Patricia, a Mexican woman, came north to Tijuana and crossed over the border by foot, along with her five-year-old son and a "coyote," or guide. During the trip she was separated from her child, and when she arrived in Orange County, California, the coyote extorted an additional $300 before he would turn the child over to her. Rosa, an illiterate Guatemalan woman from a rural hamlet, mortgaged her little plot of land for cash when her husband became very sick. Alone, she walked across the border to Mexico and literally hid behind bushes during the day. At night, she walked north and secured a second-class bus ticket in a rickety bus until she reached Tijuana. Then she paid a coyote to help her cross the border. She suffered additional traumas, including hunger and fear, until she arrived at a friend's home in Southern California. Throughout all this she knew that if she did not send money back home to Guatemala to pay off her debt, she would lose the small parcel of land she owned as well as her house.

Favazza (1980) describes the phenomenon of "sojourning," which is a brief and voluntary exposure to new cultures. This tends to result in fewer and less severe adjustment problems for the immigrant, since the sojourner is there temporarily only to earn money and then returns to his or her homeland. In fact, a study reported in the *Los Angeles Times* (Knight, 1997) showed that many immigrants return home after a ten-year period. "Settling" is a more permanent type of migration through which the individual, either voluntarily or on a forced basis, accepts aspects of the new culture. Favazza argues that migration by itself does not generate psychiatric vulnerability. However, prejudice toward immigrants, especially those individuals with darker complexions, may cause low self-esteem and self-hatred.

Immigrants often are engulfed by waves of nostalgia and unrealistically glorify their homeland. Typically these are men and women who leave their families behind, or who are single and plan to return home. Such nostalgic individuals experience depression and oversensitivity, irritability, and a tendency to aggression. They may have sleep disorders and gastrointestinal problems. Often, they experience role confusion and psychosocial disorientation as the consequence of having been uprooted from their own culture. If they are refugees and fearful of returning home, they may experience more stress (Verdonk, 1979). Generally, immigrants to urban areas experience more stress, particularly in terms of goal striving, as they seek to better themselves economically and socially. They have higher rates of mental illness than their rural counterparts. Housing problems can create additional stress for them. It is not uncommon for ten to eleven people to be jammed into a small, two-bedroom apartment. Guadalupe is a good example. Her husband was so devoted to his own sister who helped to raise him in Michoacán that when she and two other brothers migrated to the United States, they all moved into Guadalupe's house, taking over the bedrooms.

Racism, Discrimination, Prejudice, and Stereotypes Facing the Latino Client

Immigrants commonly experience racism, discrimination, prejudice, and stereotyping, which frequently happen to many people of color in the United States. This subjects immigrants to severe emotional strain. They may turn inward and value their cultural difference even more, taking pride in their roots and looking to their cultural heritage as a source of strength and an avenue to enhance the richness of their experience. Institutional racism often restricts opportunities for immigrants to utilize existing mental health facilities. In the county where I reside and practice, only a small number of Spanish-speaking psychotherapists are available to work in nonagency settings to meet the mental health needs of this community.

Although fewer in number, immigrants who have been highly trained and were experienced professionals in their homeland have additional stressors. Now they are obliged to accept positions that are beneath the social status which they would have enjoyed back home. Clark, fifty years old, was a lawyer in Bolivia, and handled legal affairs for well-placed bureaucrats and middle-class clients. When I asked him about differences in the U.S. legal system compared to those at home, he jokingly stated that a person needed to know less about the law in Bolivia than how much a particular judge charged in order to make the case work out to the lawyer's benefit. Yet, when he immigrated to the United States, he first sold T-shirts in downtown Los Angeles. He used up his meager savings until he went bankrupt. Then in desperation he became a resident manager in an apartment complex because he had good mechanical abilities and could fix faucets, air conditioners, and the like. He needed the small apartment that came with his job to avoid being turned out into the street.

Many, like Clark, find migration to be a devastating experience when they can qualify for a well-paid profession back in their homeland. Often, they migrate because professional salaries in Latin America are relatively low, and technology is costly wherever one goes. Their age confers few benefits in the United States compared to the way that immigrants are generally treated in their homeland. While age suggests wisdom and demands respect in Latin America, it is not at all the case in the United States.

For many Latino immigrants, it is often psychologically demeaning to be confronted with a youth-oriented culture where parental authority over children is challenged. Many men and women are appalled by the lack of respect their children show them. The children are often sullen and resentful of their parents' "old-fashioned ways." Youngsters often find adjustments to a new country easier to make, although the customs and cultural heritage that were valued back home may be in conflict with their new surroundings. Young people often see American personality characteristics as more desirable than their own, and they may denounce and reject their own cultural background.

Less educated immigrants face numerous handicaps such as language problems. If they cannot understand and speak English, they are at a disadvantage, and one of their children may be called upon to interpret and relay messages for them. They miss out on what is happening all around them. Feelings of paranoia, suspicion, distrust, and dependency often follow. In work environments, immigrants who are unable to learn English or who do not have not the skills to study find themselves passed over for promotion, which causes them to feel helpless and discriminated against. As Seligman (1975) has argued, cognitive, motivational, and affective problems follow from constant experiences of helplessness.

Immigrants often miss the sense of community that they left behind. For example, Nestor was desperate to return to Mexico, although his wife was greatly opposed. He claimed that he could not stand the noise of an urban environment and the alienation of urban life. He missed the *rancho,* and despite the life opportunities for his children in the United States, he was adamant about returning. All his life he had depended on his extended family, who were no longer available to him in the United States. Life crises that the immigrant experiences such as sickness, death, marriage, birth, and unemployment in these instances must be faced by the individual alone.

Immigrant Social Networks

Overall, we can see how immigrants are at a great risk of developing psychiatric illness as the result of their migratory experiences. The process of cultural bereavement, whereby groups of people suffer permanent traumatic loss of their familiar landscape and culture, is not uncommon (Helman, 1994). Some evidence suggests that Mexican immigrants do have smaller interaction networks than subsequent generations, and they are more likely to rely on their family for emotional support. Legal immigrant households are more likely to be multigenerational in nature. Researchers have found that the longer the family stays in the United States, the more likely they are to reunite with family members who, in turn, immigrate from Mexico, and the more likely they are to have children born in the United States. The family becomes binational with the passage of time and the birth of native-born children.

Immigrants maintain a strong emphasis on social and family ties. Most immigrants, even if they arrive legally, know many others who have come to the United States illegally. The geographic proximity of the United States to Mexico and Central America means that immigrants often return to their homeland and reenter the United States on different occasions. Border cities such as Tijuana and Mexicali are easy to visit, if one's documents, such as a passport, are in order.

Immigrant adjustment often means that immigrants who leave their homeland and who are severing personal ties that gave meaning to their lives will suffer a loss. There is empirical evidence that some immigrants who express this sense of loss are likely to experience depression (Vega, Kolody, and Valle, 1987). Recent epidemiological studies, however, indicate that standardized rates of psychiatric disorders and distress, including depression, are no higher among Mexican immigrants than within nonimmigrant populations (Moscicki et al., 1989). In 1995, Fabrega wrote that the availability of social resources in the receiving nation may be the distinguishing factor in the social adjustment of the immigrant. There is certainly a need for resource and information assistance. One of the major roles of the psychotherapist is as an information specialist and psychological educator to alert clients to resources for whatever problems are most pressing.

In the anger management groups that I conduct, I find that men and women who end up in the criminal justice system generally have very small social networks. Whatever networks are available are used primarily to accomplish the actual immigration process. Support within these networks facilitates the acquisition of basic materials and existential requirements to survive in a new country. In short-term therapy that generally emanates from employee assistance program referrals, the psychotherapist has the most opportunity to link the clients with community resources and increase their interactional network as it relates to the particular psychological issue involved.

COMMUNICATION STYLE

The psychotherapist in managed care must find a way to make a quick assessment of the client without using tests or scales, given the time constraints involved, to discover the most beneficial approach to take in working with the client. Communication style is the first variable of importance. Is the client monolingual in Spanish? How long has he or she been in the United States? Does the client or the children speak English? If so, how fluent are they?

There are numerous dialectic differences within each Latin American country, as well as different curse words and obscenities. When I lived in Peru and traveled with my then-fiancé to Chile and Argentina on vacation, in both places we carried letters of recommendation to friends of friends. When we arrived in Santiago, and later in Buenos Aires, my fiancé and the men in the group sat down in a serious manner. The first order of business was not to inquire after the health of our mutual friends, but rather to review curse words in the language of each country that we would not necessarily know about, which might not be acceptable or polite. For example, if I want to talk about diet with a rural Mexican laborer, instead of using the word *huevo* (egg), which in some circles is the slang word for testicles, I would be better advised to use *blanquillos* (little white ones). A sign of the client's acculturation in the United States is the extent to which he or she handles compound or borrowed words such as *los biles* (bills to be paid) instead of *las cuentas, el truco* (the truck) instead of *camion,* etc. Bilingual therapists, too, find themselves code switching—changing language in midstream. In many family sessions with parents, children, and adolescents, the psychotherapist often speaks Spanish to the parents and English to the children in the same sentence. This is especially true when the therapist is involved in negotiating behavioral contracts. This code switching is a factor that adolescents generally appreciate, as they often pride themselves on their English skills and may feel more comfortable speaking English rather than Spanish.

Nonverbal communication is also very important to consider. Anthropologists write a good deal about contact versus noncontact cultures. Latin Americans are very tactile compared with Anglo-Saxons. Handshakes are a must, even with children and certainly with their parents. As a sign of class membership, one finds that upper-class and middle-class women often shake hands in a limp manner, although it can be quite subtle. That can be a clue to their education, class aspirations, and value systems. As a woman, I often give an *abrazo* (a formal hug) to a woman whom I have just met, after spending an hour listening to her really difficult life problems, abuses, losses, etc., especially if any type of catharsis occurs as the result of her ability to unburden her secrets. It is not unusual for me to be expected to kiss an elder female as a sign of caring, although, again, I may not know her very well. Certainly, counselors are obliged to self-disclose in order to create more reciprocal relations with clients (see Triandis et al., 1984). For the psychotherapist trained in psychodynamic theory, this can be a very uncomfortable activity and even can be viewed as undermining the goals of therapy.

ETHNIC IDENTITY AND VALUE ORIENTATION

Another important variable to recognize is the client's ethnic identity and value system. It is important to know where clients were born, how long they have been in the United States, and how closely they identify with their ethnic group. A fair number of clients speak English poorly, yet nonetheless they may at first wish to speak to the therapist in English, simply to show that they are just like everybody else. These clients often revert to Spanish when they need to talk about emotional issues.

If the client has an unusual surname, in a language such as Nahuatl or another Native American language, it is appropriate to comment on the name. I find that my own surname, Rios, acquired in marriage, enables me to talk about how some names are so common (Rios means rivers), while other names, such as the client's, may not be. On several occasions I have noted a Portuguese or French name, which indicates some family history. For example, the Emperor Maximilian left a number of French soldiers behind on his retreat from Mexico in the nineteenth century. They fled to the hills where they lived quietly for many years, intermarrying with Mexican women. A Mexican laborer from Nayarit with a Huichol Indian surname may have suffered additional humiliation, perhaps branded as an *indio* (Indian) in his own country and treated disparagingly. These identity issues may contribute to understanding the clinical picture better, especially concerning personality disorders.

Respect *(respeto)* toward elders is still an important value, and the family's well-being is often viewed as more important than that of the individual. I will look at collectivist versus individualistic concepts of the self in Chapter 4. Latino families prefer nurturing, loving, intimate, and respectful relationships. Immigrants often bring to their new destination the same complex social class squabbles and prejudices that they maintained in their homeland. Depending on the degree of mestizo heritage and history, they make invidious comparisons with others who may be more darkly pigmented than themselves, or who bear American Indian or African physical characteristics, although one encounters little institutional racism.

Simoni and Perez (1995) have argued that the underutilization of mental health services by Latinos may be due to the incompatibility of psychological services with Latino cultural values and characteristics. Simoni and Perez also focus on the concept of power distance—the extent to which a society affirms the existing power differentials between certain groups or individuals by promoting deference and respect toward powerful others. These authors find that Latinos in fact come from power-distance cultures deriving from the Spanish conquest of the New World, and they tend to value conformity and obedience, and support autocratic and authoritarian attitudes from those in charge of organizations or institutions. Related to this is the trait of lineality, which stresses the role of authority in the solution of problems. Status within a hierarchical structure, thus, is important. For the clinician, this translates into the importance of symbolic clues in office decor, personal dress, visibility of framed degrees, etc., to inspire confidence in this hierarchical structure.

Another important cultural value for Latino clients concerns disclosure by the psychotherapist to create a more reciprocal relationship with the client. Although a therapist might hesitate to have a family picture visible in the office, personal items, discussions of where you grew up, a similar problem in the life of someone you once knew, etc., do create a certain sense of sharing that is well-received.

GENDER ISSUES

For every macho man who presents for therapy, there is a woman who falls into the reciprocal category of *marianismo*. This term refers to the self-sacrificing, long-suffering woman who receives a certain satisfaction from her life circumstances because she is assured of a "cloud in heaven" for her self-abnegation or martyrdom. Maria was the most extreme case of martyrdom that I had ever seen. Married to an abusive seventy-three-year-old man for many years, she had watched over the years as her husband favored one of her daughters, who stole a large sum of money from her. Despite a history of beatings and verbal abuse by her husband, and alienating one of her daughters, Maria nursed her husband as he lay dying of cancer, at great personal expense to herself. She left home only to go to early Mass each day.

Gender issues need to be examined in light of changing cultural patterns. The concept of machismo is not exclusively Latino by any means but is widespread among lower socioeconomic groups throughout American and European society as well (Gilmore and Gilmore, 1990). Data from low-income Anglo groups reveal the same type of male dominance that the term macho brings to mind. Major value is placed on a man's ability to be a good provider, and men fear not working because of illness or injury. Depression, anxiety, or panic disorders are seen by men as a sign of weakness or mental illness, and not congruent with their status as strong men.

Some writers have seen Latino machismo as a cult of virility, arrogance, and sexual aggression of men toward women, although the concept of responsibility toward the family also exists. As the result of acculturation, traditional expectations appear to be changing. I rarely see exaggerated machismo patterns in couples who come for help within the managed care setting. There is a frank recognition and pleasure in the wife's earning capacity and how her economic help can contribute to the maintenance of a middle-class lifestyle.

Claudia was a good example. She and her husband were both of Mexican Indian background, living in Southern California, and suffering from economic problems, including bankruptcy. Claudia was incapacitated with a panic disorder and agoraphobia, ever since she had been caught by the Immigration and Naturalization Service and sent back to Mexico. Her inability to leave the house and work to supplement her husband's income was a major stressor in their marriage.

Interdependence of spouses seems to be more common among couples in counseling, at least when both spouses work. In some cultures, however, the cultural framework in which men are traditionally socialized validates their masculinity through control, power, and competition (see Castenada et al., 1996). Pleck (1981) argues that men who are unable to live up to these traditional demands of a man's life can experience role stress and are more likely to engage in high-risk behaviors such as consuming alcohol and drugs in excessive amounts. Or they may exhibit outbursts of violence toward others, or be promiscuous and engage in unsafe sex. This is particularly pervasive in the modern world where machismo, overall, is on the decline as the result of economic advancements, equal protection of women under the law, and, for many Latinos, acculturation (Comas-Diaz and Greene, 1994).

When we look at the sociodemographics of Latina women compared to other immigrants in the United States, we see that Mexican women have the lowest educational levels among Latinas. This leads to high levels of unemployment and poverty. Early socialization stereotypes these women and fails to equip them with skills and competence, which in turn undermines their self-confidence and can lay the foundation for mental health problems in adulthood. Such women lack confidence, have a tendency to blame themselves when things go wrong, and do not take credit for success (Vasquez, 1994). Depression, anxiety, and trauma responses are commonplace. There

is a real need to teach the client assertiveness skills, conflict management, and strategies of positive self-talk.

Latina women are socialized differently than men. Men are seen as
entitled to have their needs met without regard to women's feelings,
while women are socialized to feel responsible for the well-being of
others. Women assume blame and responsibility for failure or for
negative, painful experiences. The psychotherapist must not encourage Latina clients to adapt to unhealthy environments but rather
empower them to change those environments or leave them behind.
There is a need to emphasize the client's strengths rather than weaknesses, to validate her worth and to send her a clear message that she
is responsible for her problems and only she can cause positive outcomes for herself and her children.

Latino family structures have to be differentiated as healthy and
functional on one hand and dysfunctional on the other. Healthy families demonstrate a mutuality and respect for ascribed roles. The
working father and homemaker mother do not preclude equity in
decision making and conflict resolution. By contrast, in dysfunctional families, as Vasquez (1994) points out, traditional roles are
carried out in an oppressive and pathological manner, with power
battles, abusive behavior, poor conflict resolution, and low marital
satisfaction. In such families, Latina women internalize their expectation to nurture, care for, and maintain family unity and connections.
Often, the woman may be in denial or ignore her own needs in her
attempts to keep the family intact even when her husband is abusing
her. Vasquez (1994) presents statistics about violence against Latinas,
which is an issue of concern. Wife abuse is found in all social, economic, religious, ethnic, and educational levels, from 26 to 60 percent incidence for all couples with a higher incidence of wife abuse in
lower socioeconomic classes.

A woman's identity is partly based on the messages that she
receives from significant others about herself. Among many Latina
immigrant women, we find restrictive gender and sex-role stereotyping from early childhood on, which often fails to equip girls with
skills and competence as well as undermining their self-confidence.
This may lay the foundation for mental health problems in adulthood.
Racism, especially for mestizo-looking individuals, can lead a woman
to feel badly about herself. A positive aspect of Latina gender, how-

ever, is Latino familialism and the support a woman can generally expect from her family members. It has been suggested that the individuation process, which is an important therapeutic issue in Western psychotherapies, proceeds differently for Latinos. Values for females, such as independence, individuality, and competition, may be different for Latinos than for their American counterparts.

Bem's (1981) gender schema theory argues that individuals become sex typed and acquire gender-appropriate preferences, skills, personality attributes, behavior, and self-concepts very early in life. Children are cognitively ready to encode and organize information about themselves in accordance with their own culture's definition of masculinity and feminity. A child born into a traditional Latino family where male and female roles are very strictly defined is in turn socialized to assume his or her respective gender role. This sex typing is a learned phenomenon and often changes under acculturation pressure. For example, several female clients have come to me to complain bitterly about their daughters, who appear very masculine to their Latina mothers. These older women, socialized elsewhere, are appalled that their daughters are not wearing pearl jewelry or other trinkets as a badge of feminity.

The traditional male gender scheme thrives in more stable agrarian environments, where the male head of the family is expected to maintain control of his emotions and provide a sense of security and stability (Casas et al., 1994). Such a man is the final arbiter of significant decisions within the family and is the source of economic power. The wife takes care of the family and is in charge of household responsibilities. What works in a stable environment in rural Latin America may not be very useful for an immigrant family in the United States, where male gender schemas that are now maladaptive are challenged. I see this every week in anger management classes that I provide for court-mandated clients, where Latino men tell me they must confront any challenge to their masculinity, despite the consequences.

It is not at all unusual to encounter situations in which a single mother with several children works a night shift to get higher pay. Josefina not only left her sixteen-year-old son alone while she worked, but left him in the charge of her second husband, who was only ten years older than the boy. The two fought uncontrollably and Josefina could not understand how neglected and cast off her son felt.

Octavio Paz (1980), noted Mexican poet and writer, in his book *Labyrinth of Solitude,* directs our attention to Cortés's mistress, Malinche, who in the sixteenth century bore the Spanish conqueror an illegitimate son. Often seen as the source of Latin American society's misogynist attitudes toward women, Malinche is a symbol of the mestizo "race"—the individual who possesses both European and Native American heritage. Malinche played an important role in Cortés's conquest of Mexico, and the duality of female existence that Paz portrays in the Mexican character—the saint/whore—would have Malinche at one pole and the Virgin of Guadalupe at the other (see also Castenada et al., 1996).

Marianismo—the cult of feminine spiritual superiority—is the reciprocal of the Malinche figure. Perhaps the exaggerated makeup of the *chola* or gang-girl seen in some Mexican-American barrios is a rejection of the saintly, self-abnegating female martyr, who has an infinite capacity to experience humility and sacrifice. Women according to the value system of *marianismo* are seen as morally superior to and spiritually stronger than men. Although machismo may exist, Latinas, as others elsewhere have done, turn to covert manipulation power tactics as a strategy of the oppressed. The submissive wife can actually be the one who, by acting helpless, manages whatever happens in the marital relationship.

The area of machismo that spills over into the courtship and conquest stage often takes the form of *piropos,* which are verbal expressions said by a man to or about a woman in her presence. Directly or indirectly, this talk comments on her physical attractiveness. Some *piropos* are negative and demeaning to women, focusing on the dual image of the woman as both harlot and virgin. The custom originated in southern Europe and found its way to Latin America.

One can see a link to machismo here in that the Latin American male child develops an intense attachment to his mother and the world of women, especially the children I see who are highly indulged—*consentido*—with a nearly unconditional love, resulting in an intense and personal relationship. This leads to a high degree of protectiveness and outright encouragement of dependence. In agrarian-based families, the child suffers a serious blow at the birth of the next sibling, as it is not unusual for a farming family to desire ten to twelve children. A new baby can lead to a trauma and abrupt weaning from the previous indulgence.

Some writers such as Suarez-Orozco and Dundes (1984), with a psychoanalytic bent, argue that the Don Juan syndrome develops as a primitive attempt at mastering this first loss by the male child who is engulfed in an early mother-son symbiosis. The father is generally aloof and emotionally remote from the child. Once the boy begins to associate with older males and the father, he is ridiculed and accused of effeminate behavior—a potential homosexual—since he has spent all his time with women. The child then moves from a privileged existence among women to a submissive position in the world of men. To become a man, he has to make a drastic break with the female universe and submit completely to older males.

Suarez-Orozco and Dundes argue that this initial period of over-identification with the mother and Latino males' excessive concern with being masculine lead to a denigration of women and are the core of machismo. The child's difficulty in identifying with the male figure creates profound doubts in the boy about his sexuality and his general adequacy. Hypermasculinity—macho behavior—and ambivalent emotions toward women may be the central outcome of this dilemma. The child's hatred and rage toward the mother for expelling him from his idyllic existence before the birth of his sibling, these authors believe, causes a displacement to women generally and a reaction formation of viewing the mother as a virginal angel. The *piropos,* especially the negative ones, are outlets for men to ventilate the ambivalence of their emotions toward women.

Domestic Violence

If Suarez-Orozco and Dundes (1984) are correct in their formulation of the machismo complex in its negative aspects, then domestic violence issues cannot be far behind. Sociological studies on violence against women, in general, have neglected the plight of the Latino female. Kanuha (1994) points out that ethnic minority groups are overrepresented in the use of public services such as emergency rooms, community health clinics, and other social welfare programs and, thus, are overrepresented in indices of negative social conditions such as poverty, crime, disease, child abuse, and domestic violence.

Thorne-Finch (1992) has argued that violence is a manifestation of both individual psychopathology and learned behavior with roots in early childhood abuse, family dysfunction, and drug abuse or disorders of personality, thought, or impulse control.

Since early 1973, there has been a shelter for battered women in our county. Sullivan, a graduate student of mine, studied this shelter, which housed thirty-seven Hispanics, of whom twenty-eight were Mexican nationals. When compared to Anglo women in the shelter, the Latinas had a lower socioeconomic level, were married longer, and were more likely to tolerate abuse. The Latina women seemed to experience certain acts of violence more frequently before they would consider them abusive. Mexican women in shelters tended to marry younger, stay married longer, and have larger families.

Sullivan found two types of abuse, major and minor, which included pushing and shoving in the minor category, and broken bones, bruises, etc., in the major category. The Latinas studied more frequently lacked economic resources, which made it difficult for them to leave an abusive relationship. The Latinas also had more children than their Anglo counterparts, which was the main reason that the Latinas were more likely to leave their abusers. They were more likely to call the police. The median age of the abused women in the shelter was twenty-six years compared to thirty-three for Anglo-Americans. Latinas worked in low-paying, low-status jobs and had lower median incomes. More of the Latina families were headed by women. Among the Latinas in the shelter, there was a high fertility rate, which mirrored national statistics overall, with 28 percent of Latino births in the United States to unmarried mothers compared to 11 percent of Anglo-American families. Ninety-four percent of Latino women had battering partners who used alcohol; 52 percent also used illegal drugs such as cocaine and marijuana. As many as 30 percent of clients in this shelter were Mexican nationals or from Latin America. The Latina women placed high value on keeping the family together, especially when children were involved. Many of the Latina women who were victims of violence commonly had also experienced violence in their family of origin. Typically as girls they were discouraged from being assertive or independent and they were socialized to be passive and compliant. They suffered from low self-esteem and had difficulty in self-validation. Many were sorely in need of conflict resolution skills due to their limited education.

As Kanuha shows, a number of sociocultural factors affect battered women of color. Latinas are reluctant to bring attention to themselves, their families, and their communities for fear of contributing to the stereotyping of people of color as pathological. Ethnic stereotypes argue that women of color are stalwart and resilient in the face of all odds. Some Latina women ascribe the causes of domestic violence to the influence of organized religious doctrine, particularly Catholicism, upon the attitudes and behaviors of men toward women. Gender roles of men and women in Latino cultural groups not infrequently delineate the complex expectations and responsibilities of men as superior and honor-bound, and females as passive, compliant, and responsive to others' needs (Ginorio and Reno, 1986).

Acculturation explains any important variations in understanding when women define their rights in terms of the degree to which they are assimilated to the values and practices espoused by Westerners. One battered woman, Elsa, whom I visited in her relatives' home a few days after she was released from the hospital after being knifed by her husband, told the victims-of-crime official working on her case that they should not waste any money sending a counselor to meet with her as she was worthless. This woman was a recent immigrant and had not learned anything about women's rights in this new setting in which she found herself. Therapists working with Latino immigrant populations should not expect a high level of knowledge about laws concerning women's rights and must exercise their educational function as well.

Bem (1981) has shown that there is a cultural framework in which men are traditionally socialized to validate their masculinity through control, power, and competition, which in turn encourages or validates their violence. Alcohol is important in that it helps such men to overcome societal proscriptions against emotional expression, especially between men. There may be a male gender-role need to feel omnipotent that can be temporarily satisfied by alcohol, drugs, or excessive sex. Certainly machismo is not a solely Latino phenomenon, as it is found in most cultures worldwide. Among the Latino population, this phenomenon is widespread.

The strong relationship between self-esteem and gender identity helps to explain why traditionally oriented Latino men are reluctant to relinquish extremely macho beliefs, attitudes, and behaviors, which can contribute to the development of serious mental and health-related problems for themselves and/or their families.

If a family emigrates to the United States, the change of environment significantly challenges the male gender schema that was adaptive in a previous setting but now is maladaptive in the current situation. Many families I have counseled tell me that the father only began being abusive and drinking to excess after emigrating from Mexico or Central America. Back home, he would only get drunk on a holiday or special occasion. These macho men are not likely to seek therapy where they will appear as helpless or weak and where they will no longer be in control of their situation. Generally women initiate the process and threaten to leave to get their men into therapy.

Casas and colleagues (1994) suggest that clinicians must intervene in ways that remove some of the internalized barriers that impede traditional male clients' access to the therapeutic process, by focusing on the wounded self-esteem and lack of motivation of men forced to admit their inability to cope with their lives and who have to seek help from others. Casas and colleagues suggest that the therapist has to reframe his or her statements to argue that a truly strong person is one who can acknowledge difficulties and obtain temporary assistance to surmount them. It is thus in the client's best interests to do so. Classes rather than personal counseling are viewed more favorably by men. Not infrequently, adherence to the masculine gender role may lead to somatization of emotional problems, and men in this group will not attend to physical symptoms or medical conditions since to do so would betray the schema of male strength and invulnerability.

CULTURAL MORES

The therapist needs to pay attention to the client's customs in his or her home country. Is the patient devoutly Catholic? If suicidal ideation is present, what are the culturally appropriate arguments that the psychotherapist can use to minimize the possibility that the client will ever consider taking his or her life? Is the client a member of a charismatic or spiritist church *(espiritista)* that encourages dissociative behavior? This can be important for the therapist to understand if he or she is diagnosing and treating a patient who may enter a trance state. If so, do trances occur within a formal religious context, as opposed to being independent, peripheral responses by the client? The basic premise behind spiritism is that good spirits will reward people with their protection. The psychotherapist, needless to say, is obliged to respect the client's religiosity, even if such beliefs are contradictory to his or her own. Even a persuasive skeptic such as psychologist John Schumaker (1995) agrees that religiosity and good mental health go hand in hand.

David's wife, Esmerelda, however, carried her spiritual concerns a little far. For her, the espiritista church in Puerto Rico where she was a devotee, along with possession by spirits, helped her deal with her near-psychotic dissociative states. When she kidnapped her four children and ran off to Hartford, Connecticut, with them, David was very upset and took a leave of absence from his job to follow her. He, too, was very devout and prayed over me for my well-being at the termination of each clinical hour.

How does the client's religious tradition treat issues of death and dying? The resolution of grief? What are the client's beliefs about eschatology, that branch of philosophy which deals with life after death? Many health professionals themselves are not comfortable with the religious beliefs of others. Yet, we must be careful not to dismiss other people's beliefs as delusions when these beliefs emanate from a religious identity. Although I am not myself involved with any formal religious structure, on the rare occasion when asked, I tell my clients that I am a *simpatizante* (sympathizer, one who respects traditions), although I am sure that this can also create some discomfort. On occasion, clients will proselytize and try to get the therapist to show an interest in attending a religious service in their church.

Other areas of importance include sexuality. Many clients have never heard the term "orgasm" and women may not have experienced sexual pleasure. It is not unusual to suggest sensate focusing exercises for married couples who complain of sexual dysfunction. For the immigrant woman catapulted into single or premature parenthood, low income, or multiple jobs, a focus on intrapsychic conflicts might be wasteful of her time and energy. The therapist needs to act as a social worker, to ameliorate some of the stressors in her environment to ensure a more effective therapeutic intervention. Often the therapist must try to change the family structures within the socio-cultural and ecological context, rather than focusing on individual behavior. Therapy must be of short duration, oriented to the present, and focused on concrete problem resolution and mobilizing the family and the individual to cope more effectively with stressful life situations. Another issue facing single mothers has to do with the need to feel comfortable in assigning tasks to their children to help them around the house, including their growing sons who can easily handle their own laundry once they can operate the washing machine.

HEALTH BELIEFS AND PRACTICES

Health beliefs and practices vary tremendously among Latino immigrants. Although such men and women may have insurance, their managed care plans differ tremendously with regard to the prevention education that they make available, especially in Spanish. Often due to time constraints or English language deficiencies, the client may not be given much explanation of the health problems he or she faces unless the primary care physician is bilingual and takes the time to educate the client. Elia, a single mother with four children who was accused of child neglect is a good example. She lost her child for a few months to foster care. The hospital where her three-year-old daughter was being treated for hypothyroidism reported her to the county's Child Protective Services. According to the client, the nurses, who spoke poor Spanish, miscommunicated to her the seriousness of her daughter's physical problems and how important it was to give the child thyroid medication. The child's abnormal blood levels led doctors to the conclusion that the mother was neglectful of her daughter's well-being.

One of the important functions that a psychotherapist fills is to talk about mind-body integration and holistic health, the integrating of good diet, exercise, healthful lifestyle issues, and health and mental health attitudes into a life plan that makes sense for the client. I find myself frequently explaining how the body works and how certain medicines function. I keep nearby in my reference bookcase authoritative pill books on the effects of the medications that the client is taking for high blood pressure, ulcers, orthopedic problems, etc. Whenever possible, I utilize metaphors to make the client understand how the body works.

Even something as simple as blood pressure is news to many clients. People are quick to remember their actual blood pressure readings, both diastolic and systolic, but in many cases, no one has ever bothered to explain that the heart is like a pump. I physically imitate a pump pushing and then resting, pushing and resting. If the bottom number of a client's blood pressure reading is too high, I say that the heart is not resting, and that the valve can fibrillate. I illustrate this with my hands waving in the air. I say that this can result in a fatal heart attack if not promptly responded to. Many of my Latin American clients who lived in great poverty in their homelands now have the income to increase the amount of red meat in their diets. It is not unusual to find clients eating meat in all of the week's twenty-one meals, plus snacks. It is important to explain the concept of cholesterol to those who do not understand the relationship between diet and heart disease.

Beliefs in herbalism and folk healing are commonplace among immigrants. Clients turn to local health food shops or *botanicas* (herbal shops), which dot the Southern California landscape, to find their hawthorn berry potion for irregular heartbeat, which is available in a tea. Often these brews can be quite potent. Any psychiatric evaluation must determine whether such potent plants are being ingested by the client. Popular literature suggests that 150 herbal preparations readily available in health food stores may indeed have psychoactive properties.

A good example of herbal medicine "gone wrong" is the case of Nélida, who came to see me with a severe depression. When I asked her, as I do all my clients, what other herbal medicines she might be using, she listed seven or eight major plants such as *valerian* that I knew to be psychoactive. When she stopped taking all of them at my request, she responded well to the antidepressant medications that the psychiatrist had prescribed for her and finally was able to sleep. At the sixth and last session, she admitted that she was back on valerian, but that she was feeling much better and was able to think about getting a job. Overdoses of plant preparations can precipitate adverse mental health effects, and the psychotherapist must be alert to the possibility that the client will be supplementing any prescribed medicines with home remedies *(remedios caseros)*.

Many Spanish-speaking immigrants, if not true believers in witchcraft, do originate from communities where hexes are realities for many and certainly not delusions. When I lived in the Amazon, not only were witches pointed out to me, but it was said that they had little black books and took whopping fees to harm a person's enemy, provided that the client paid well in advance. I even had a run-in with one reputed witch, who accused me of getting ready to denounce him to the authorities. Since all my water in the Amazon slum where I lived had to be brought to me in buckets, I worried for a couple of weeks that this evildoer might try to poison me. I only felt better when he left on a long trip!

Culture-specific illnesses called *daño, empacho,* and *susto* are all well known by clients. Many believe that physical and mental problems result from witchcraft hexes. Jorge, a Salvadoran man living in Los Angeles, experienced post-traumatic stress disorder in the wake of an industrial accident. He found his ex-girlfriend visiting his sister at their home when he was not expected to be there. She was placing a *cochinada* (filthy, pig-like) hex mixture of animal feces, blood, and plant materials in the corner of his closet to make him fall in love with her again.

For the clinician assessing the Latino immigrant client, cultural biases will affect DSM-IV diagnoses. They range from mental retardation and other disorders of children (e.g., reading, mathematics, written expression, attention deficit hyperactivity disorder, and conduct disorders) to separation anxiety disorders, somatization disorders, schizophrenia, and other psychotic disorders. Psychosocial stressors take on an important role for the clinician, who must be alert to language barriers, discrimination, and value conflicts, which have to be assessed in the initial phase of treatment with Latino clients. As Padilla (1994) argues, inattention to cultural factors in the diagnostic process lead to misdiagnosis and subsequent errors in treatment.

In the next chapter, I look at the psychotherapeutic techniques that are most effective in treating the Latino immigrant's mental health problems.

Chapter 3

Techniques That Work
with the Spanish-Speaking Client

From my studies of shamanism and traditional folk healing in Peru, I learned that most healers and patients often attribute the cause of illness and even misfortune to the work of malevolent spirits or other forces in nature that a psychologist would argue are simply projections of one's own feelings and anxieties upon the world at large. Insight therapies, however suited they may be for short-term interventions, in my opinion are not beneficial for immigrant clients. These individuals originate from societies where shamanic healing traditions are still part of historical memory (and where they still exist in some cases), and their attribution of causality is projected outward to spirits and evildoers. Even modern psychotherapy, as Walsh (1989) has pointed out, makes use of experiences analogous to cosmic traveling or the shamanic journey. Psychotherapists, in fact, use a wide range of imagery techniques called "active imagination" by Jung (cited in Campbell; 1973). These include visualizations, guided imagery, guided meditation, or waking dreams. I will discuss hypnosis shortly, which is a powerful technique that I find very well received among Latino clients, analogous to the shamanic journey (Walsh, 1989).

The techniques I have found to be most effective to reach the Latino immigrant population and to relieve psychological symptoms of distress are hypnosis, behavior modification, and cognitive restructuring.

Hypnosis or the use of suggestibility to effect changes in thoughts, feelings, and behaviors is very compatible with traditional folk healing. For one thing, the psychotherapist/hypnotist must be a high-status person, just as the healer is a respected member of the community. Part of therapists' presentation of self must include highlighting what is important and noteworthy about themselves and their accomplishments. Diplomas on the wall certainly are indicated. While many of the urban poor may have as little as three to six years of formal schooling, they do understand the reality of class structures in Latin America, where education is a prerequisite for the wealthy, powerful, and successful individual. As Simoni and Perez (1995) argue, Latin American society indeed supports clear-cut differences between certain groups or individuals by promoting deference and respect toward powerful others—the wealthy, the aged, and those in prestigious professions. Latinos come from a high power-distance culture.

THE SOCIAL STATUS OF THE THERAPIST

When I conducted fieldwork in the Amazon, I wore gold earrings, a gold bracelet, and rings each day. This was not because I wanted to show off my possessions, but rather as a symbol of high social status. The concept was that if I were an important person, I was worth befriending. During the colonial period, the typical responsibilities of the large landowner *(haciendado)* included a role for his wife, clearly in a different social category than the laborer. Her charitable duty was to care for and protect the estate's peasants and their families. The idea that the doer of good deeds would be earning credits in heaven, enshrined in Catholic doctrine, is fully understood by many Latin American peasants. Indeed, in seeking baptismal sponsors for their children, such men and women commonly cross social class lines and ask wealthy patrons to stand up for newborn children.

This historical factor can be applied in a health care setting, where psychotherapists generally come from different social strata than their clients. As long as the more powerful person is viewed as being under a moral obligation to help the less powerful, a comfortable reciprocal relationship can be established. I always make sure that my clients know I am affiliated with a regional university. That presumed wisdom helps me to be direct with clients as I attempt to intervene in their lives. Frequently, as an afterthought and during a final visit, a client will bring in a teenage child so that I can provide career counseling as well. Spanish-speaking clients are likely to pay attention to friendly, high-status individuals whom they encounter in a helping role, similar to their expectations in the social world they left behind. When I lived in an urban slum in the Amazon, my fiancé and I were asked to be godparents on several occasions, since it meant that we had to buy the child's clothing and pay for the beer and food that inevitably accompanied the occasion. Once when I was godmother at a first communion in a rural agricultural village in northern Peru, I was shown a lively goat being held down by the villagers and then had to watch as its throat was cut before my eyes. About two hours later, I had to smile as I ate my portion of the cooked meat!

GENDER OF THE PSYCHOTHERAPIST

Sometimes in dealing with immigrant clients, questions arise about the gender of the psychotherapist. Should the therapist be the same sex as the client or not? Of course, in some cases when a man's sexual dysfunction may be at issue, it is perfectly natural that he may not wish to discuss his sexual inadequacy, penile dysfunction, etc., with a woman if he believes that this will shame him in some way. In managed care settings, however, the client may have little choice about the sex of the therapist, especially if the language issue means that fewer psychotherapists are available. People tend to make do. If the psychotherapist has techniques that can help the client, gender issues often become irrelevant. That does not mean that the psychotherapist should be unaware of the discomfort that the client may experience. One way to deal with this issue is to use a shamanic technique—namely in terms of self-presentation. It often is useful to state one's own qualifications with regard to the clinical issue. My monologue to a patient might go as follows: "I have seen many cases like your own, Mr. X., and I have a long history of helping others with similar problems." Many of the traditional healers with whom I worked in South America were quick to provide their clients with a summary of their wondrous deeds.

When I was studying rural folk healing on the coast of Peru in the summer of 1967, I remember Don Ricardo, who had a thriving healing practice in a small town called Salas. At sunset, as the patients were getting ready to assemble in a nearby field where his healing ministrations would take place, Don Ricardo was complimented by his clients on the warm alpaca poncho that he was wearing. During the session, he looked me in the eye and said in a loud and boastful voice, "Do you like this? Isn't it great? It was given to me by a patient whose illness I cured." Everyone was suitably impressed. A few weeks later, on my way back to California, I stopped over in New York to visit family. I called on a well-known psychiatrist, who was interested in cross-cultural issues, at his Park Avenue townhouse. It was replete with a Zen garden and four large original Picasso paintings on the wall. I was suitably impressed. I always wondered if there was any real difference between the two healers, as both presented themselves in a positive manner, in the symbolic language of their respective cultures.

Another technique with shamanic overtones concerns clients who come into short-term psychotherapy either agitated with sleep disturbances, or with appetite loss. The technique derives from the insights of Mauss (1973), a nineteenth-century social scientist. In his book, *The Gift,* he wrote about the process of gift-giving and the reciprocal relationship it establishes between recipient and donor. Beginning in 1982 when I first began to work at the Burn Center at the University of California, Irvine, I developed a culturally relevant hypnotic relaxation tape, which I give to almost all of my clients who exhibit any symptoms of pain, anxiety, or depression, or who suffer from sleep disturbances. The tape makes use of the high-tactile focus of Latino cultures and suggests that energy is to be moved slowly into the client's body, from the top of the head to the shoulders, to the tips of the fingers, to the chest and the back, to the waist, to the knees, and finally to the toes. The tape describes restful scenes of beaches or meadows. It asks clients to see themselves sleeping peacefully at night, all night long in their beds, having wonderful dreams. The tape makes a heartfelt, inexpensive gift that the psychotherapist can give to a client. Once the client receives the tape, he or she is instructed to listen to it two or three times a day and before going to sleep. The client often experiences symptom relief. Although he or she may not expect to pay the psychotherapist for the tape, the client does feel morally obliged to return to the second appointment. In all societies, one always recognizes a gift-giver. Perhaps there may be other valuable gifts in store!

I purchase large numbers of inexpensive cassette tapes and duplicate the relaxation exercise both in English and Spanish. I make a fuss about offering a tape as a gift, which I say is "especially for you." This is resonant with the first theme of *personalismo* in Latino cultures, where dignity and personal qualities of an individual are valued, recognized, and honored in social interactions. High value is placed on a person's inner attributes, characteristics of self-respect and dignity. Such a valuation is more important than the economic or social status of an individual—the result of a caste system established since the European conquest. The cost of cementing this reciprocal relationship is quite minimal—about seventy-eight to eighty-five cents as a business expense for the cost of a tape.

A second theme on the relaxation tape that I find advantageous is a metaphor of empowerment to enhance the client's self-esteem, which I intersperse throughout the tape. The client is likened to a wonderful eagle, king of his dominion. The image is based on an ancient legend in Toltec history. These people left their homeland in the north of Mexico in prehistoric times and settled in Tenochtitlán, central Mexico. According to an often-repeated prophesy, they ended their journey when they found an eagle perched on a cactus plant, holding a snake in its mouth. This emblem, in fact, is represented on the Mexican flag and is a meaningful symbol even to those without much education (de Rios and Friedman, 1987).

Relaxation tapes are of practical benefit to clients who need to control pain due to burns, orthopedic or neurologic injury, or migraine headaches. The tapes are short and to the point. Text can be added to the tape as needed, with suggestions and metaphors to meet the specific problems that the client faces. These additions are discussed further in Chapter 4, when I look at particular clinical problems that clients have and the appropriate metaphors to call upon to meet their needs. Appendix A presents the text of the tapes in English and Spanish, so that psychotherapists can make their own gift of healing to their Latino clients.

Behavior modification techniques are helpful for parents who have difficulties dealing with their minor children, many of whom are becoming Americanized too quickly for their parents' taste. These techniques also help clients deal with family and work issues. I explain psychological principles in Spanish, particularly the concept of reward and punishment. A gift of a "good kid" chart (see Daily Duties, Appendix B) is offered to parents, who are asked to make copies for each week and are shown how to negotiate contracts with their children. Writing contracts between children and parents may be a novel experience for many uprooted peasants, now living in cities, whose personal memories are of stern parents who rarely played with them as children, or who took little time to explain and reason with them when they misbehaved. Nonetheless, most people recognize a good thing when they see it. Kids in particular catch on quickly to the inherent benefits in such contracts for themselves, such as more outings, trips to theme parks, treats, etc.

To the children, I explain principles of negotiation. I use the metaphor of a vendor of a fine Arabian horse, who demands $200 for a horse worth $100. The buyer offers $25 for the horse, knowing full well its value. Then, each side bargains further, with the seller lowering the price to $150 as the buyer offers $50. Finally, when both parties agree to a $100 selling price, everyone is happy. The buyer knows that even though he has asked $200 for the horse, he has gotten the full value of $100. The seller is pleased that he was able to bring the exorbitant price of $200 down to the true value of the horse, namely $100.

In many Latin American poverty-stricken environments that I have studied, commercial activity is highly developed, as people survive economically by buying and selling items, to which they add a small markup. This commercial concept can easily be generalized to negotiation with children and parents in order to achieve a balance and harmony in everyday affairs with which all parties can live. In this case, writing contracts and posting them in visible places such as on the refrigerator provide parents with serviceable techniques that are effective interventions. The Systematic Training for Effective Parenting (STEP) program for parents in Spanish can be purchased by the psychotherapist in bulk (see Appendix B) and resold to parents at cost. The system teaches ways to discipline and deal with a child's misbehaviors in a nonviolent and rational manner. This intervention can be labeled "acculturation education." Adlerian concepts such as understanding and implementing the logical consequences of a child's behavior may not always be acceptable to Latino parents, who themselves often remember a strict childhood where they learned to acknowledge that their parents were always right. Now, parents are suddenly expected to act democratically and to allow their children to negotiate for their rights. I inform parents that outcomes are what counts, and I instruct children to continue to show signs of respect to their parents so that they, too, can achieve their goals.

A third helpful technique is cognitive restructuring, although it must be adapted to a client population that boasts little formal education. Many of my clients read and write very little in their leisure time. If they do purchase the STEP program, I suggest that the husband and wife read a chapter aloud and discuss how they can implement the principles in their own home.

Although cognitive techniques such as journal keeping, written logs, and diaries are used effectively by psychologists in clinical practice, they are not particularly applicable to people who possess little schooling. Because of poverty and the lack of schools in the Latin American countryside, clients respond much better to rhetorical, verbal techniques such as those found in rational-emotive therapy (RET). These techniques can be helpful to alleviate psychological distress and discomfort. I use one of the RET diagnostic tests for irrational beliefs, which I have translated into Spanish to help me evaluate rapidly what some of these irrational beliefs are (see Appendix B). This permits me to develop a dialogue with clients, to help them confront their irrational beliefs and to discover just how they are being held hostage by their own thinking process. Confronting irrational beliefs is a challenge, and it can take one or two visits to work through the test results. At this point, the psychotherapist can easily introduce proverbs and sayings to challenge the client's irrational beliefs, particularly with regard to self-acceptance and frustration. Thus, for example, the saying "I'm not a golden coin that jingles happily in everyone's pocket!" *(!No soy monedita de oro para caerle bien a todos!)* is a good way to deal with the irrational need that some people have to be liked by everyone, all the time, without fail.

Most of my Spanish-speaking clients read few books or magazines, and they seldom write letters in the age of telephone links to even the most rural outback. A certain percentage of clients go to school to learn English, although many who have been in the United States since 1987, the cutoff year for amnesty, speak little or no English. Nonetheless, everyone knows how to take a position on an issue and, to different degrees, to verbally defend their point of view. The psychotherapist has to be very gentle in the process so as not to appear too confrontational. The gentle prodding of a client's irrational beliefs can produce some real insight for people who may have grown up in dysfunctional families, perhaps with an alcoholic or violent parent present, who took little time with them to explore different options in problem solving.

Within the tradition of cognitive psychology, it is important for the psychotherapist to teach clients to resolve problems, to explore different options available to them, and to reach a rational decision based on clear and level-headed thinking. Poor people have clusters of problems. For example, many individuals have poor math skills due to their limited education. A large number of my clients do not know how to do long division, a skill learned in the United States in the fourth or fifth grade. Some uneducated people are naturally talented in mathematics, but it is common to find people, even when they have two incomes in the family, taking on mortgages whose monthly payments represent 60 to 70 percent of their gross earnings. One can imagine the scope of these clients' economic problems. Far too many go bankrupt and lose their homes. One of the skills acquisition training tasks that is helpful for the psychotherapist to provide is to prepare a monthly budget so that clients can see that they truly are "in over their heads." Those who have large credit card debts need to be referred to nonprofit, state-supported credit counselors to help them reduce their debt load.

When I lived in Peru, one of my university colleagues there had problems buying a small house. She had to pay 35 percent of the cost of the house for the down payment, and then pay off the mortgage in five years' time. This is not uncommon in Mexico and elsewhere in Latin America. In the United States, by contrast, clients who are employed often have easy access to credit. With the numerous credit cards that are readily available to them, clients often overspend. In the last year, I have treated at least six clients who owned expensive time-share condos in resort areas, and numerous others enrolled in expensive fitness programs, although they could hardly make ends meet each month. They fell victim to hard-sell sales pitches despite their lack of resources. The temptations of credit cards are great, as Latino families are very generous with their children and often find it hard to deny their children toys, clothing, and outings, which again results in overwhelming credit debts.

Credit liability can create problems, too, for battered women or unhappy wives who want to separate from their husbands. As a main concern, these women often worry about losing their credit. While the role of the psychotherapist is certainly not that of legal adviser, it is imperative to understand some of the basic principles of bankruptcy and contract law. A book called *La Ley y Sus Derechos* (The Law and Your Rights), with bilingual Spanish and English text (see Appendix B), is a smart purchase for clients who know very little about business law. By the same token, I find it important to instruct clients about how the IRS works and why it is important to be honest and direct in general in dealing with governmental agencies.

In Latin America, there is a wonderful saying: *"Si tiene enemigo, aplícale la ley!"* (If you have an enemy, apply the law to him!). As anthropologists have long since realized, in many societies with agrarian traditions where kinship bonds are preeminent, one must make a business colleague into an esteemed friend so that morality will triumph and contracts will be kept. Latin American justice systems may not enforce contract provisions in a meaningful way. By the same token, bureaucratic salaries are often unrealistically low, and it is often expected that bribes will supplement bureaucrats' salaries. Under these circumstances, Latinos learn not to take rules too seriously. Thus, the Latino client with middle-class aspirations who may now be an immigrant in the United States can only assume that what is true at home is true everywhere. Far too often, clients have to extricate themselves from conflicts with a variety of agencies such as the Social Security Administration, the IRS, or the INS because of outright lies they told after they were advised by the people around them to put their best foot forward even if the details were exaggerated or untrue.

Denis was a good example of this. He suffered for a long time with bipolar disorder and found many reasons not to pay his state income tax. After three years he received several letters from the State Franchise Board, which demanded that he file. I gave Denis's wife the names of two reputable accountants who specialized in tax law. Later, the wife told me that Denis was irate that the accountant he selected was not interested in anything but a straightforward response to his liability. What? No tricks?

Another skills technique helpful for Latino men and women is assertiveness training. There is a real problem for the psychotherapist in translating the word "assertive" into Spanish. One has to use another term, such as appropriate positive self-presentation, to approximate the concept. I have found it invaluable to create a Spanish-language handout that compares passive, assertive, and aggressive behavior. I also train the client to state messages in an assertive manner, to avoid blaming others and to express personal feelings directly and succinctly. Assertiveness training is particularly helpful with depressed women who are involved in bad marriages with traditional Latino husbands who demand that their wives behave the way they did back home in their rural community. Such assertiveness training can reduce stress for Latina women whose husbands may attempt to overcontrol their every move or thought. Appendix B presents an assertiveness chart in English and Spanish that the psychotherapist will find helpful in his or her practice.

Bibliotherapy is a fairly common intervention with upper-middle-class and middle-class Anglo clients. Psychotherapists often recommend good reading to help clients understand the patterns of their lives and how their particular clinical issues may be part of a larger social pattern. The type of bibliotherapy that I conduct with the immigrant client is somewhat different. The main technique is analogy. Thus, when after two or three sessions a battered woman admits to being knocked around by her boyfriend, lover, or husband and is frightened to leave the home because of the children, I am likely to extract from my nearby bookcase a book by a noted psychologist. I tell the client (it is actually hearsay) that this person was a consultant on the O. J. Simpson trial because she was such an expert. Then I provide a loose translation from the book concerning the pattern of wife battering. Often, the client identifies with the three-stage scenario of tension building in a household, battering, and then a period of romantic reconciliation. Women begin to recount their own experiences as they reflect this pattern. At this point, it is much easier to make a meaningful intervention, such as getting the woman and her children out of the house and into a shelter or to seek protection elsewhere before any more blood is shed.

As with the shaman, psychotherapists must establish the validity of their credentials so that their interventions are more readily accepted by the client. When people come to me and tell me of suggestions to solve their problems from people whom they know casually, I tell the story about the donkey who was taken to market to be sold. As the story goes, a man and his wife are taking their two young children to a market some five towns away to sell their donkey. In the first village that they come to, the people stand around in the street and scold the man for not riding on the donkey. So he mounts up. In the second village another person scolds the man for making his wife walk while he rides. So the owner allows his wife to mount the donkey as well. In the third village yet another passerby scolds the owner for letting his eldest boy walk. So the child mounts up. In the fourth village a passerby laughs out loud that the poor little girl is made to walk. So she is lifted up to ride on the donkey's back. By the time the family arrives at the fifth village where the market is located, the donkey drops dead. It does not take a formal education to get the message: Who are you going to listen to, anyhow, and how good is his advice?

To summarize the benefits of cognitive-behavioral therapy with Latino immigrant clients, three fundamental ideas are applicable to all populations: (1) cognitive activity affects behavior; (2) cognitive activity may be monitored and altered; and (3) desired behavior change may be effected through cognitive change (Lewis, 1994). The cognitive structures that function as templates to guide our perceptions and interpretations are cultural constructs, and as Beck and colleagues (1979) have pointed out, dysfunctional schemata give rise to negative thinking patterns. Culture can exacerbate irrational beliefs, especially when it sets up extreme and impossible-to-achieve norms. Lewis (1994) addresses concerns of Latina women of color and delineates stress-inducing beliefs that are developed by women in the sex-role socialization process. They include the need to be loved and approved by every significant person in a woman's life; that other peoples' needs count more than one's own; that it is easier to avoid than to face life's difficulties; that a strong person is necessary in life to lean on or to provide for one; and that women don't have control over their emotions (Fodor, 1988; Wolfe and Fodor, 1975). This therapy approach is helpful in combating the damaging effects of a paternalistic system that can emanate from the machismo/*marianismo* system found throughout Latin America.

What makes these techniques so special? In the next chapter, I will talk about metaphors in general and how they can aid the psychotherapist who treats Spanish-speaking patients. I will also look at insights from a newly flourishing field called cultural psychology.

Chapter 4

Metaphor and Misery: Does Everyone Think the Same Way?

Short-term therapy for the Latino immigrant patient is strongly dependent upon cognitive restructuring to relieve symptoms and to heal the misery the patient experiences. Insights from medical anthropology can help us understand the nature of cognitive differences, if any, between people who originate from different cultures. This is especially true in situations where Western-style education is minimal, and metaphor, proverbs, and other symbolic and analogic techniques form the basis for an individual's decision making and comprehension.

Before looking at the metaphor as a linguistic tool to communicate, it is important to examine the question, Do other people think differently than we do? In the postmodern era, over the past fifteen years, there has been a growing awareness that so-called reality is truly the construction of those who believe they have discovered and investigated it. Anthropologists such as Shweder and Bourne (1982) argue that many ideas and practices among human beings fall beyond the scope of deductive and inductive reason. Rather, ideas and practices can be said to be neither rational nor irrational but nonrational, or symbolic. Much of our action says something about what we stand for. Our nonrational constructions of realities come from stories and give us frames of reference through which we grasp at reality. Shweder and others are interested in differences between cultures and in how the individual's distinctiveness is partially informed by cultural factors.

We must be careful not to fall into the trap of the early evolutionist social science writers, who were committed to the idea that other ways of thinking are less adequate stages leading up to the development of our own understanding. Clearly, European and American society are not the endpoint of human development. As Shweder and Bourne (1982) argue, there is no way to say whether one form of understanding is better or worse than another. Cultural relativists try to preserve the integrity of the differences between people and to establish the coequality of varieties of forms of life. Shweder and Bourne would have us seek and obtain as much information as possible about the details of other people's way of thinking, their symbolic system, the meanings they ascribe to life—"the native's point of view"—so that we can see the sense of their beliefs and conclusions.

As psychotherapists, this information can help us to treat our clients effectively. Much of this nonrational belief falls beyond the scope of scientific evaluation. It is only the evaluation of the individual functioning as a member of society that provides the positive or negative value for his or her belief or action. Shweder and Levine (1984) call this "cognitive egalitarianism," which gives the psychotherapist a moment of pause when responding to cultural patterns that may appear abnormal in light of his or her own cultural background. We will see considerable variance between cultures when we look at marital issues that occur with Latino immigrants. There are also other value-conflicted issues that the psychotherapist must confront in his or her own culture that may not sit comfortably when dealing with Latino immigrants.

The relativist position also has its problems. Other people's understandings are said to be self-contained in people's own ideational universe, and there are no common standards across cultures. However, immigrants who acculturate to a different world, one that is also in flux, must adapt to this new environment in order to survive. Powerful messages come to them through the media, from the schools that their children attend, and from their work environment.

Javier's run-in with the legal system is a good example of this. He worked as a skilled laborer at the same factory for several years, and he was proud of his good relationships with his co-workers. One day he was in a good mood and gave an *abrazo* (hug) to a woman co-worker with whom he thought he had a joking relationship. As he recounted the story, he put his left arm around her shoulder and his hand rested just below her upper chest. The woman reported him to the human resources department for sexual harassment and sued him, which resulted in his arrest and presence in an anger management class. *Abrazos* are common in Latin America between men and men, or women and women. Javier thought he was being "cute" or flirty, to show off his manliness. He learned a costly lesson indeed!

Cognitive differences between individuals from different cultures are often pointed out. Evolutionary theorists see these cognitive skills as unequally distributed across cultures and even as deficits. Many argue that abstract classification is a wholly alien procedure to some people. Can we argue that schools, in general, foster a person's ability to abstract, to generalize, and to think scientifically? Can we say that people are concrete thinkers in their adaptation to a rural lifestyle that is different from that of urban civilizations? Are such people less likely to reflect on alternative cultural practices or, in contrast, to see their own customs and beliefs in a more general comparative framework? What about informational limitations on people's lives when they live in a world that lacks literacy, urbanization, and external influences? Critics of this approach, however, point to the world of storytelling, metaphors, and analogies where different cultures use distinctive abstract systems that are conceptually uncalibrated but equally present in all cultures. Thus, there is no simple intellectual equivalency standard that can be used to compare two cultures. In fact, Shweder would argue that in no culture can any conceptual system encode all possible relationships and abstractness between truths. All systems are concrete and abstract at the same time.

Cole's (1996) early study of Mexican peoples demonstrated clearly that schooling brings about fundamental changes in a person's cognitive development. Implicitly or explicitly, children learn cognitive tasks such as deliberate remembering, formal reasoning, and logical syllogisms. People who have no schooling, by contrast, look to "empirical plausibility." Their guiding maxim is "practice makes perfect." Piaget and others agree that in cultures without formal schooling, formal operational thinking does not develop. Shweder and Bourne (1982) argue that the best model to understand the cognitive development of the individual is not to view the person as an information processing system. Rather, human beings inhabit intentional worlds and find meanings and resources from their sociocultural environments.

Shweder is a relativist who argues that the concept of the person has to be seen in a larger whole that relates the individual to the society. Many evolutionary theories view schooling as a prerequisite to abstraction skills. However, the fact that people react with insight and delight to symbols such as metaphors, proverbs, and stories shows us that skills of abstraction simply take on a different form. Shweder argues that cultures differ less in basic cognitive skills such as generalization and abstraction than in the metaphors by which they live, the hypotheses that people build about the world they live in, and the ideas that underlie their social action. All people are perfectly competent to process information, and they can differentiate, generalize, and take on the perspectives of others. However, they often place little value on these activities or on differentiating people from their social roles. These intellectual moves are unimportant to them as their worldview directs their attention and passion to particular systems.

COGNITIVE DEVELOPMENT AND SCHOOLING

Metaphors are valuable and quick methods to communicate in order to enable patients in psychotherapy to develop their own solutions to their problems (Berlin et al., 1991). Any metaphor that is based on clients' personal experiences and perceptions as well as deriving from their culture is likely to succeed. This tool is very useful in the short-term treatment of a client because the psychotherapist does not have to patiently explain his or her own explanatory model to the client, to convince the client to value scientific experimentation and data-gathering techniques, etc. Metaphors can be used as teaching tools, as part of the psychoeducation that any psychotherapist must provide for the immigrant client. The metaphor is a means of therapeutic communication and can motivate clients to achieve therapeutic change without having to change their explanatory models of reality simply to please the therapist. Lankton and Lankton (1989) argue that clients are less resistant to metaphors in psychotherapy because they are nonconfrontational ways to consider change. The metaphor is a story that does not require any response but simply stimulates thinking and experiencing. These traits are necessary for problem resolution. Dolan (1986) sees a metaphor as a road map. A good metaphor provides the client with a comprehensible and quick map to resolve problems. Metaphors stimulate the client's own inner resources, memories, dreams, goals, fears, and hopes, especially if they are well chosen and reflect key elements of the client's problem as the client searches within for the appropriate meaning.

Anthropologists have been curious about the different styles of thinking that have characterized different peoples of the world for many centuries. We can go back in recorded history to the writings of a Greek, Herodotus, who noted that the Egyptians were different from the Greeks because they kept cats as house pets! Recent studies show that people may not think the same way, that indeed they organize their realities differently. Linguists are aware that language often categorizes the universe. Infants who learn the meaningful sound units or phonemes of the language spoken by their family and community will map out that universe long before they actually experience it for themselves. Immigrants originate from tribal nonliterate societies of Latin America as well as from societies where Western education has made few inroads (e.g., people with three or four years of primary education, with rote learning, who grew up in a rural setting, without television, telephones, or mass media), or among the urban poor in anonymous, massive squatter settlements in capital and provincial cities throughout Latin America. People there may be dependent upon examples and analogies as learning tools. Rhetoric, storytelling, mythologies, and legends, recounted in song and ceremony, have a real impact in learning. For the psychotherapist who works with a clientele of individuals who have had little formal schooling, the ability to tell stories and recount proverbs and *dichos* can make an impact on the client beyond what he or she imagines.

Siegelman (1990) sees metaphor as the way that we come to understand the world. Metaphor is a way that we construct the world we live in through our perceptions. For Siegelman, the metaphor is a process in which a person describes one thing in terms of another, so that a third thing, a new idea, is born. We can argue that it is a basic property of the mind to seek analogies. The metaphor is evidence of abstract seeing that uses concrete sensory experience. Thus, the visual conveys abstract ideas. The abstract is arrived at through the concrete, by use of the senses. Metaphor is useful to bridge or to generalize so that thought can cover a larger domain than it originally did (Kopp, 1995). Metaphor connects with the world that people sense and feel (Grove, 1989). Moreover, metaphor is similar to hypnosis in that it engages all the senses—visual, gustatory, auditory, and kinesthetic. For immigrant clients who have little formal training, this concrete style of experiencing lends itself very comfortably to the use of metaphor.

Since managed care psychotherapy with Latino immigrants is time-limited, the therapist is obliged to generate the metaphors. By using specific metaphors from folklore, myth, or fairytales, a metaphoric image can be introduced by the therapist to teach or illustrate a psychological problem. The psychotherapist has to guide the client. In fact, we can think of people's lives as stories and work with them so that they experience their life stories in ways that are meaningful and fulfilling (see Freedman and Combs, 1996). These narratives are guiding metaphors. An anthropologist might put a particular spin on this by trying to get inside the person's head, understand his or her culture, and then use that knowledge to help the client. By using cultural wisdom encapsulated in proverbs and sayings, we can help people to reinterpret their experiences and find new solutions to their problems.

The enlightenment position in Western thought holds that human beings are intentionally rational and scientific. The so-called dictates of reason are equally binding for all people, no matter when, where, or what their culture, race, or individual abilities. Reason is said to be a universally applicable standard to judge validity and worth. Any culture that distances itself from this Western ideal was seen to be backward or primitive. In contrast, Stigler, Shweder, and Herdt (1990) view ideas and practices that have their foundation neither in logic nor empirical science and which fall beyond the scope of deductive and inductive reason as nonrational. This would include presuppositions, cultural definitions, arbitrary classification, and probably metaphor. Nonrational constructions of reality come from stories and provide us with frames of reference to grasp reality. Howard (1991) talks about different frames that present differing views of reality to people, with the idea that no frame is superior to another.

Clients tell therapists their life stories, and therapists obtain an idea of clients' orientation to life, their goals and ambitions, and pressures that surround the presenting problem. The therapist can only wonder if the problem is a minor deviation from an otherwise healthy life story, a normal, developmentally appropriate adjustment issue. Or, more complex problems may be going on. If the life story is problematic, then a rebuilding effort may be necessary. Howard (1991) argues that the work between the client and the therapist is a life story elaboration, adjustment, and repair. As we will see in Chapter 6, different metaphors can be part of this process.

In order to communicate clearly and meaningfully to people whose life experiences may have been different from one's own, the psychotherapist must employ metaphors that arise from specific social contexts of agrarian life when interacting with immigrants from rural backgrounds. This is particularly germane to ensure communication success for pain control (which I discuss in Chapter 6) and to convey an understanding of surgical procedures for patients and in other medical contexts.

Using metaphors in psychotherapy is hardly new. Several recent books focus on the importance of metaphor in psychology. The use of figures of speech in which a word or phrase is applied to an object or action that it does not literally denote in order to imply a resemblance is probably the basis of much traditional healing communication (Mills and Crowley, 1986; Zuniga, 1991). There are indeed multiple levels of communication between people. Freud (1953), in his book *The Interpretation of Dreams,* showed how metaphor and pun play a major role in psychic processes. Metaphor has an important role in behavioral techniques because it can capture the imagination and inspire people to undertake tasks or think about things in a new way that they may not otherwise do.

From a psychoanalytic perspective, metaphors often are used to analyze patient material or to make interpretations. However, in short-term psychotherapy, the psychotherapist has little luxury to slowly derive metaphors from client productions the way that long-term therapy might permit. Rather, the psychotherapist needs to use a generative metaphor, one that creates a new way to understand a problem and to derive a possible solution. In this way, situations that at first seem complex and uncertain become clearer. A new metaphor, especially if it makes a person laugh, creates a new logic for solving the problem and renders new meanings and ideas for new actions (Berlin et al., 1991). Unlike the psychoanalytically derived metaphor, which takes longer to obtain and which emanates from the client's wellspring of experience, the metaphors I discuss in this book are external to the individual. They resonate with his or her culture and carry personal meaning. The metaphor can simplify an idea by emphasizing certain elements in a different way. Like computer software that allows us to highlight an issue, we can then reframe the problem in a new way to disrupt a previously held idea or behavior.

Berlin et al. (1991) argue that metaphors are playful and serious at the same time. They allow the therapist to communicate highly personal aspects of the patient's behavior without appearing intrusive. Metaphors are affectively charged and equate two dissimilar subjects. Patients must acknowledge their own assumptions and contributions to their difficulties. Interestingly enough, the metaphor emphasizes a relationship between situations and not a particular set of facts. The patient who does not have much schooling can make the abstract leap easily through imagery.

Using metaphor to confront a client's misery yields benefits. It is important to understand that the background and educational attainments of the Latino immigrant client will determine the degree to which metaphors will be a powerful communication tool to enhance treatment success. The sayings that I find most helpful to use with clients can be placed in different problem categories. They include statements for couples in therapy, for anger management, for acting-out adolescents, for cognitive restructuring, for acculturation education, for masochistic women, for grief counseling, and to motivate depressed men and women to set goals and to act on them.

METAPHORS: SOME EXAMPLES

For the suffering wife who receives little affection or attention from her husband, the phrase *"A la mujer ni todo el amor ni todo el dinero"* (Give your wife neither all your love nor all your money), helps her realize what a short leash her husband has her on, and why she feels like she is choking. For example, when Elazar's common-law husband wanted her to marry him to enable him to obtain immigration documents even though he was legally married to another woman in Ecuador, she knew that if she acquiesced, she would become a party to bigamy. This was in addition to other mistreatment that she was suffering, including insults and his occasional pushing and shoving her. She considered leaving him. The client responded to the phrase *"Al que le duele la muela, que se la saque"* (If your tooth hurts, you should pull it out).

Arnulfo and his wife, Alina, had a different problem. Impulsive and outspoken, Alina was quick to point out her husband's numerous faults, which only led to shouting and loud arguments. While I was trying to teach effective listening and feedback skills to both of them, I told Alina, *"En boca cerrada no entran moscas"* (Keep your mouth closed so you won't stick your foot in it).

A major marital theme that I see, especially among older Spanish-speaking clients, is the unhappy wife, verbally abused, ignored, and mistreated for many years, who refuses to leave the husband and is afraid to live alone, unprotected. The saying *"Lo que no se puede remediar hay que aguantar"* (What can't be remedied has to be endured) is often reassuring.

Leonor lived with her husband for more than thirty years. He was a workaholic with a small business. He rarely came home until late and was verbally abusive to her and their two grown sons, who worked in his manufacturing plant. Leonor managed to endure her isolation and neglect by developing a parallel life. She spent time in church activities and with family members. Her revenge was to develop ailments and pains that few doctors were able to treat successfully, although she spent her husband's money going from one clinic to another. The saying *"Tanto bajo el cántaro al agua hasta que se quiebra"* (The ladle dips into the water so much that it finally breaks) was helpful to her. This metaphor enabled Leonor to understand the enormous stress she was under and how it adversely affected her health.

Working with Spanish-speaking, court-mandated clients who have run afoul of the law because of their anger can be very challenging to the psychotherapist. The workbook that I use for anger management is full of cognitive exercises to help clients learn to modify their thought processes when they are provoked by irritating people or situations. The *dicho "Antes de hablar es bueno pensar"* (It's a good idea to think before speaking) reminds them that when they are quick to tell people what they think of them that a moment's reflection may be in order before they act. The *dicho "Cuesta poquito mas para vivir en paz"* (It costs a little more work to live in peace) can clarify the futility of speaking one's mind just to get a word in edgewise without evaluating the consequences.

Foolhardy, angry young men are frequent visitors to these groups, including José, who got into a car fight with another driver who made an obscene gesture as José cut him off. The two battled it out, ramming each other's cars until the other man stopped and both started screaming at each other. José punched in the wing window of the other man's car, then jumped back in his pickup and fled the scene. His license plate was duly noted. After he spent a week in jail and paid a fine, he was sent to the anger management program. The adage *"El que no agarra consejo no llega a viejo"* (He who doesn't listen to good advice will not live to old age) made an impression on him, as he was the father of two young children, and he was motivated to learn to control his anger.

Gonzalo was also in the anger management group and had a different kind of problem. Illiterate, and from a small village in northern Mexico, he had an unpleasant run-in at a fast-food chicken restaurant where he paid for two plates of food for his wife and himself. Although he was given a receipt to claim his food, he told the group that he threw it away because he was unable to read it. When his order of food arrived with only one plate, he began to argue with the server and finally threw the plate of food at him. The food was splattered all over the floor and the clerk. Gonzalo was arrested and was told never to darken the restaurant's door again. The saying *"No des un paso sin ver para atras"* (Look before you leap) was helpful to him on a subsequent occasion, this time in a different restaurant. When he became angry, thinking that he was being cheated, he remembered the adage, the court fine, and his forced attendance at classes, which made him reflect and sidestep a second incident.

Elogio, too, had trouble controlling his anger and sought out men his age to provoke them to fight with him. According to him, he never got into trouble until an incident when he was suspended from work for starting a fight. He came to psychotherapy due to an EAP referral. Typically, he said, he would provoke the person who annoyed him (e.g., a man got in front of him in line), until the other man struck the first blow. Then he would spring into action, down his opponent, and punch him out. He responded well to the saying *"Quien ama al peligro en él perece"* (He who loves danger will perish in it).

When I try to show anger management clients ways to right injustices and to resolve problems without resorting to fighting or name-calling, they tell me about bullies at home, at work, or in the market who insult them and make their lives miserable. I try to help clients see what other options and alternatives are available to them so that they can "win" in a peaceable manner. The *dicho "Tambien para los pinos hay hacha"* (Even for pine trees we find axes) is useful—that is, the idea that even a large pine tree can be felled, meaning that a major problem can be overcome.

It is helpful to use the RET model as a cognitive-restructuring technique to help clients become more flexible in their approach to life and to relinquish their sense of catastrophe and disaster if things do not happen as they expect. Telling the client that *"No hay rosa sin espina"* (There's no rose without a thorn) is a good way to counter the perfectionist stance of the rigid man or woman who must have everything turn out a certain way. I also point out that "The deafest person is the one who does not want to hear" *(No hay peor sordo que el que no quiere oir)*. In fact, when trying to convince a client that it is okay when not everyone in the world esteems him or her, or that it is not so terrible or horrible to make a mistake when someone is looking, I say that "Even the best cook can ruin the meal" *(A la mejor cocinera se la ahuma la olla)*. Clients who are quick to see catastrophe loom in every problem they encounter are angered when incidents occur that are unjust and unfair. They recognize the truth of the saying "Money talks" *(El dinero lo puede todo)*—that is, it is not a fair world, especially when they have had difficulties with the criminal justice system and have not had the money to hire a lawyer or to learn how the system is structured. When clients insist on perfection from themselves and others, the *dicho "El hombre propone y Dios dispone"* (Man proposes and God disposes) is welcomed.

When parents and their adolescent child disagree about the value of the adolescent's friends, the child often is not in a position to understand why Mom or Dad is fearful about exposure to gang activities or lack of adult monitors in the friends' families if they are dysfunctional. To the parents and often in the presence of the adolescent, I quote the saying *"Dime con quién andas y te diré quien eres"* (Tell me with whom you go and I'll tell you who you are). Two other similar sayings are helpful in alerting parents to the dangers of giving in to their teenagers, who may not be mature or experienced enough to make a good decision: the phrases *"Pajaros de la misma pluma vuelan juntos"* (Birds of a feather flock together) and *"Dios les crean y ellos se juntan"* (God creates them and they find each other).

There are some *dichos* that I find myself repeating again and again because of their applicability to many clients who have troublesome friends or relatives. The first one, *"La leña enseña,"* literally translates to mean that firewood teaches. Patients often have experiences with recalcitrant spouses or children, when it appears to them that nothing they have done or will do can change the behavior of a significant person. If the psychotherapist has to come up with suggestions and interventions that can be described as "tough love," the *dicho* makes good sense here. That is, as you know, with some folks, only *"La leña enseña."* Often this may give rise to an elusive flash of insight, the "Eureka!" phenomenon that motivates people to try a new technique (e.g., negotiating with a teenage child, getting a battering husband to stop, etc.). Nonetheless, clients do understand the principle, which may be quite abstract, although the analogy is very concrete. I imagine that if I were hit over the head with a piece of firewood, it would be quite painful, but certainly effective in getting my attention.

In these instances, I tell a story that I read in a local newspaper some years ago. I try to be dramatic in the telling because, as a practitioner who models her techniques on shamanic performance, a dramatic edge is expected. I modulate my voice, with high and low registers. I hesitate at the punch line so that the message comes across well. The story goes as follows:

> One day a circus came to town and everyone was amazed to see a donkey jump through a ring of fire. The local newspaper reporter went out to interview the trainer to learn his secrets with the animal. In the dressing room, the trainer said, "I'll be happy to show you how I make the donkey jump through the ring of fire, but let's go outside for a demonstration." With that,

the trainer picked up a heavy beam of wood that was lying on the floor and was about to go out the door. The journalist asked him why he picked up the beam and was told to come on out and see for himself. Once outside at the spot where the donkey was tethered, the trainer smacked the poor donkey on his backside with a powerful blow. The indignant journalist asked why on earth he did that, to which the trainer replied, "The first thing is—you gotta get his attention!"

While at first blush this story involves cruelty to animals, parents of teenage children react quickly to this message and are then quite receptive to my suggestions for ways to get the child's attention, such as grounding the child, limiting telephone privileges, confiscating clothes left on the floor for a few days, etc. In agrarian environments with high levels of poverty, animal rights are often not a high priority.

Another story that I frequently tell when I introduce techniques of cognitive restructuring is that people often make themselves miserable because of their tendencies toward catastrophic and excessive responsiveness to the world in which they live. I ask them if they have ever heard the story of Chicken Little. I even ask those individuals who are not in the habit of reading bedtime stories to their children or who may not even have many books in their home because *cuentos de hadas,* or fairy tales, are known in every culture, and people respond well to fairy tales if they illustrate a point. This can make the acceptance of the psychotherapist's intervention more likely. As the story goes, Chicken Little was hit lightly on the head by a falling acorn. She ran and told all the animals that the sky was falling. Quickly she instructed the other animals to tell everyone! Clients are quick to laugh at the story, especially as I wave a brightly colored stuffed chicken at them, but it remains an effective way to talk about the dangers of treating everything as a catastrophe, with little reason to do so. The story leads comfortably to explanations of rational-emotive techniques that challenge the client's irrational beliefs and negative self-talk, all of which create the misery that the psychotherapist works hard to eliminate.

When I ascertain that clients have no intention of returning to their home country and see their future in the United States (this is especially true among immigrants who are legally able to work and live in the United States), I stress the need to learn English, in order to obtain marketable skills. I provide information about the educational system available to them in the region. The adage *"En la tierra a que fuiste, haz lo que viste"* (When in Rome, do as the Romans do) is quite applicable.

This discussion of proverbs, adages, and stories makes no attempt to be complete. Many of the excellent Spanish-English dictionaries have long lists of proverbs that can be adapted by the psychotherapist for particular client needs. In the next chapter, I look at a time frame for work with the Latino immigrant managed care patient and give the reader the opportunity to think about where these proverbs and stories might best fit.

Chapter 5

The Typical Course of Therapy with the Spanish-Speaking, Time-Limited Patient

As with all short-term interventions, the psychotherapist must use time wisely and take full advantage of any telephone conversation involved in making appointments. Once the referral is received (and insurers will differ in the amount of clinical information they convey verbally or in writing), I generally try to make the first telephone call. Some managed care companies prefer that the client initiate the call to the psychotherapist, but, frankly, this is counterproductive. It is hard enough for the Spanish-speaking immigrant to open up and talk to a stranger without having to initiate the interaction. By making the telephone call, I set a certain caring response in motion. This initial call also makes it possible for me to gather assessment data even before I meet the client. The therapeutic alliance, moreover, is nurtured by the client's perception that I have shown the initiative to make the first contact.

In giving directions to the office, the psychotherapist often can set down the ground rules, e.g., that it is imperative for the client to call if he or she cannot attend for some reason, or else there will be no second try. Psychotherapists must cut their losses. A certain percentage of clients (as high as one in four in all managed care referrals) do not appear for the planned initial visit. Clients who know that they will lose a subsequent opportunity to meet are more likely to reschedule a missed appointment when clinical issues are pressing. Many clients simply come one time to tell their story, never to return. I estimate that to be the case with about 20 percent of the individuals whom I see each year. The psychotherapist also must pay attention to the quality of the language interaction on the telephone. Does the client converse in the Spanish of an educated person? If not, is it hard to understand him or her? Often, when I call the client back on subsequent occasions, I may speak to a number of different people in the household—other relatives or roommates—who may answer the telephone, or there may not be an answering machine, which generally indicates a no-frills environment in this day and age when inexpensive answering devices are ubiquitous.

Ideally, the psychotherapist should have a waiting room close to the office. Often, immigrant patients will bring along their children, another child or two whom they are baby-sitting, and a spouse or parent. Children become tearful and cranky when they are left in a distant waiting room, even when a receptionist is present. As with all family therapy, it is often appropriate to interview parents separately from their children and vice versa. Since the working poor complain about their lack of discretionary cash to pay for baby-sitters, it is a good idea to keep a basketful of toys handy for quick retrieval and cleaning up. I purchase inexpensive card games from gift catalogs so that when I counsel a child, I am able to give the child a gift the first time we meet. The principle of gift giving applies to children as well as to adults. Many children of immigrants do not have an excess of toys available, and the gift generally makes an impression on the child even though the cost is minimal. It goes without saying that having crackers on hand for the hungry and whining child avoids disruption of the session if the child's needs are not met.

In many Latin American societies where corruption in social institutions can be widespread, people prefer to place their trust in people, not institutions. One must build up social support networks with reciprocity and cooperation, which is expected and valued (Simoni and Perez, 1995).

Forms of address and sincerity in dealing with individuals are pertinent. Terms of address generally mean that a woman over twenty or so is called *Señora,* a man, *Señor,* or a girl, *Señorita.* I am very careful about using the *usted* form of the verb (the formal "you"), and I rarely using the familiar *tu* form unless I am speaking to a child under fifteen or sixteen years of age. Before I begin the session, I fill out a brief intake form with the client present, for billing purposes. It also contains a release of information for the client to sign to enable me to communicate with the managed care company and the patient's doctors or attorney, if there is one. I take a brief minute or two to indicate that whatever goes on in therapy is confidential and privileged and that the client owns the privilege. The term *confianza,* or confidence, which I use, has a different meaning in Latin American culture and relates to the concept of in-group versus out-group affiliation. Only with people in a trusting relationship is the term *confianza* used. Again, this can add to a sense of trust and sincerity necessary to overcome resistance.

Clients must give me permission to communicate with other doctors who are caring for them as well as their insurance companies. I also inform clients that the law, in general, overrides confidentiality, and I use examples of suicide, homicide, child abuse, etc., to illustrate the point. On a few occasions, with referrals from employee assistance programs that were generated by supervisors, there have been employees who did not want to sign the release form. I make it clear that there will be no session unless they do so, and I indicate how the content of their discussions will be protected.

I fill out the intake form myself in the interest of time. I write much faster than most of my clients, and I can save ten or fifteen minutes by doing this. Additionally, I am sure to give the client my business card, since in Latin America the use of cards is a common practice. Even middle-class housewives have business cards printed to give out when they visit an acquaintance who may not be at home.

It is imperative to know where your clients originated (e.g., the name of the place where they were born and where they spent their early youth), as well as how many years of education they have. Sometimes I can estimate this from the type of job they have as skilled, semiskilled, or unskilled laborers. Anuncio, however, who came to see me for his depression, worked as a roofer, although he had the equivalent of an MA degree in plant sciences. He had also worked as a high school teacher of science in a small central Mexican city and was quite erudite. Occupations in the United States for immigrants, indeed, may not reflect their training and preparation back home. Saúl, too, was a good example of a successful businessman back in his provincial town in Nicaragua. His uncle was the chief surgeon in the local social security hospital. Yet he came to the United States to earn cash in asbestos removal work and to escape from an unhappy love triangle in which he was involved. He had a BA in architecture, yet he had a thriving business selling groceries in his home country to which he eventually returned.

Women who are housekeepers, janitors, or cooks often have little formal education. Gloria was referred for psychotherapy for her depression. She worked in a large hotel as a housekeeper. She had a bachelor's degree in early childhood education she had earned in Argentina but did not know how to go about revalidating her degree to find a job in a local school district, where she obviously belonged. With cases such as these, I offer to help clients prepare a résumé. I ask them to bring in their personal data on a subsequent visit and together we design a one-page résumé that helps them to be competitive in the labor market. In a bit of shamanic posturing, I let them know that such help with their résumé would cost them quite a bit of cash if they had to pay a commercial firm to do so. That reaffirms that I am here to help them as best I can.

Men who call themselves machinists are, in fact, often unskilled. They are generally trained or have experience with only one machine, and these can be tricky and pose safety hazards for them, given the fact that many are illiterate in English. They often have difficulty in understanding safety rules and switch overrides. Among the hundreds of Spanish-speaking burn patients I have seen over the past fifteen years, I have observed a large percentage of clients who were machinists, who were injured in explosions only a few months or weeks after they began to work in a factory. In most cases, they were unable to understand safety instructions available only in English.

Generally clients will tell their stories easily. The psychotherapist has to be careful to direct the details with appropriate questioning. Otherwise, a certain percentage of clients will tend to focus excessively on concrete details—"He said, she said, I said . . ."—and the presenting information will never end within the first therapy hour, nor will there be time for any intervention or treatment plan to emerge. I do not do a formal mental status exam, but I make note of any anomalies—motor retardation, irrational thought processes, unusual or blunt affect, etc.—that strike me. I also pay attention to the client's grammar and syntax, as well as vocabulary. Although Spanish is an acquired language for me, I do read, write, translate, and use dictionaries all the time to augment my knowledge. I find that I often know words in Spanish that my clients do not, because words with Latin and Greek origins are common to both English and Spanish. When I lived in the Peruvian Amazon for a year, there was no one in the entire city of Iquitos with whom I could speak English, so by force I learned to speak Spanish well!

Before the first psychotherapy hour is finished, I am sure to offer clients a gift of my Spanish-language hypnotic relaxation tape if they present with any anxiety, panic, depression, or agitation. I go into a little detail about the effectiveness of the tape and its relatively brief ten-minute length. I describe its function and how important the tape will be to help clients alleviate their presenting symptoms. I also review the number of sessions that are available and summarize my treatment goals. If the client tells me that his or her contract with managed care allows ten or twenty sessions, I point out that some may have to be saved for medication evaluation and treatment, should that be necessary. I tell the client that in general my goals are to see that the client gets better quickly.

Immigrants tend not to be particularly savvy psychologically. They accept the psychotherapist's word that he or she will get them through therapy quickly. In fact, it is crucial to set up an expectation of success and speed in all managed care interactions with clients. This goal can be more difficult to achieve with the psychologically savvy middle-class clients who may have had recourse to psychotherapy back home. Latin American psychological influences generally are psychodynamic in nature, and the expectations of well-educated clients may be for a long-term relationship.

The psychotherapist needs to explain how managed care systems work. Rather than being negative about the limited number of sessions, it is more effective for the psychotherapist to present an optimistic outlook that much can be accomplished in whatever the number of sessions available. I review my plan about the work ahead of us in the sessions we have. I usually give the client a rational-emotive therapy cognitive test in Spanish to complete at home if I think that his or her literary skills are adequate to the task (see Appendix B). If not, I will save the test for the subsequent session and will quickly read the questions to the client and mark off the responses.

From the beginning of the first session, the psychotherapist must be attuned to the client's possible need for psychiatric medication. With the managed care companies with whom I work, I make it a point to obtain the name and telephone number of any Spanish-speaking psychiatrist who is on their roster, and I try to establish some kind of working relationship with that professional. I do this either by telephone or in person, over a cup of coffee, to establish a team effort to accelerate the treatment of the client. If the physician is not a native Latin American, I assess his or her language skills to my own satisfaction, since a number of individuals may not bother to conjugate verbs in a foreign language, yet think they are still talking the lingo.

In this way, I can call upon the concept of *personalismo* if I need to recommend that a client take antidepressive medication. Since I have already been in contact with the psychiatrist, I can chat about the excellent credentials of the doctor who is being recommended, who is particularly excellent for the client's needs. Drawing on the concept in rural Latin American society that one's social networks are one's social capital, I may talk about how long I have known the doctor, how much we esteem each other, and the excellent care that he always gives to my clients. This kind of shamanic posturing not only reassures clients, who may be desperate for symptom relief, but it meets their cultural needs to have someone who is caring and personally involved with them to recognize their needs, even though they may be in a less important social category.

Regarding social categories, when I lived in the Peruvian Amazon and conducted research on traditional folk healing, I always wore gold earrings and a watch, which set me apart from the people whom I was interviewing. By the same token, it is foolish to try to appear to be "one of the guys" when in fact you *are* in a different social category. The information I communicate by this conspicuous display of jewelry, my white leather sofas in my Southern California office, etc., is that indeed I can help the client because I am important. My diplomas and certificates of study and professional membership are framed and displayed prominently. The symbolic message is not about me but rather that, as an important person, I have a personal interest in the client's well-being and I will work hard and use my talents and my social network to make him or her well. Perhaps my reward will be a cloud in heaven for the good works that I perform for the client, but we both know that the reward will come.

Prominently displayed in my waiting room are craft art and weavings from different parts of Latin America, which illustrate rural scenes and landscapes. I have a poster displaying an active Salvadoran volcano, which is useful in anger management classes because we can turn to it to symbolize a client's personal agitation or anger.

Many Spanish-speaking clients who see drug addicts and alcoholics in the barrio where they live may be hesitant to accept medicine to help them for symptom relief. If the client has major vegetative symptoms such as weight loss or gain, sleep disturbances, agitation, etc., I generally argue very strongly for the client to at least try the medication, along with continuing therapy for the duration of our sessions. I try to schedule sessions every two or three weeks to allow the effects of the medicine, once prescribed, to kick in. This gives me some leverage for a second or third visit to confirm any symptom relief and to allow time for the client to think about the behavior changes that he or she may have to make.

As early as the second or third session, I begin to evaluate the results of the cognitive-restructuring test. This is the beginning of our work to eliminate irrational beliefs and to try to help the client learn problem-solving techniques. Economic problems can be major stressors, and I generally review a client's economic profile. This is easy to lead into, since clients often complain about their bills and are seeking help in this area. A spouse is frequently invited to attend a session as additional problems surface. Or it may be time to have other family members, including children, come to family therapy. With children and adolescents, I explain the principles of negotiation and try to contract with them and their parents to resolve issues of neatness and order, schoolwork, friendship, acting-out behavior, etc. The parents and I sympathize that the way we were brought up as children may not be effective here in the United States and that it is going to be necessary to recognize that youngsters believe that they live in a democracy and that they, too, have rights. Parents and I talk about the importance of give-and-take negotiating, which indeed is a different approach from what they may have learned when they were children.

Once an immigrant man brings his wife and children to live in the United States, it is likely that he will stay longer than if he simply came alone for economic purposes. Nonetheless, a recent study shows that a hefty percentage of legal immigrants return to Mexico after a ten-year period of residence in the United States. Once settled in, however, immigrant women recognize the social leaps available to their offspring compared to the more rigid social stratification patterns at home along with their children's lack of educational access there. Women often are less willing to return home, even if there will be a new brick house in the rural hamlet or town from which they emigrated. As one client succinctly put it to me, "if you have to be poor, it is better to be poor in the United States than in Mexico."

Cognitive approaches to problem solving often bring prompt symptom relief to clients. They begin to see the world as less catastrophic in nature if events do not occur as they expect, as they find new solutions to minimize the stress in their environment. At least clients have new options to consider to solve their problems. It is likely that clients will continue to come for the duration of the allotted sessions or as long as necessary to achieve therapeutic goals. The psychotherapist must continue to confirm that the therapy is short term and to build up few expectations for long-term interaction. Axis II personality issues simply are not grist for the managed care mill. Transference issues, too, tend to be minimized by the brevity of the therapeutic encounter. Sessions are geared aggressively to relieve symptoms and to help clients acquire problem-solving techniques and strategies. The hope is that clients will be able to generalize their learning to any new situations they encounter.

I typically spend two or three sessions on cognitive-restructuring training in an effort to make it clear to the client that it is acceptable to feel sad, unhappy, and regretful when there are difficulties, but that the world is not about to come to an end if the house is not clean, if your daughter stays out an hour later than she should, and if your mother-in-law does not like you much. I use metaphors again and again to clarify issues, and I continue to apply new ones or seek out new proverbs to help influence my clients. When the last session occurs, the client and I often get sentimental about the progress made, offer a formal *abrazo* (a light touch on the arms) or hug, and pledge our openness to be available to interact again in the future. If applicable, community referrals are made. If I have done a good job, I am now part of that person's social capital and can expect an invitation in the future to a wedding, baptism, or other important life event.

Chapter 6

Clinical Issues

The psychotherapist working with Spanish-speaking, time-limited patients encounters diverse clinical issues across a broad spectrum. At present, there are simply too few psychotherapists to justify specialization. In other managed care cases where I provided services for non-Latinos, I have found that a similar diversity of cases crosses my threshold. This can be overwhelming for the provider who does not view this as a challenge to stimulate and provoke constant stretching of his or her talents as a stimulating and rewarding challenge. In this chapter, I look at the problems that most frequently are presented in time-limited psychotherapy. Special populations such as AIDS patients are not included in this discussion, since many insurance companies typically refer high-risk patients such as those suffering from AIDS to specialists.

Some of the materials that I cover, needless to say, reflect my own specialty in pain control and trauma over the past fifteen years, with my affiliation at the Burn Center at the University of California Irvine Medical Center, where I directed counseling and multicultural programs from 1982-1997. More than 50 percent of the outpatients were Spanish-speaking clients. The techniques I developed in Spanish with adult and child burn and injury patients can be applied to the short-term, Spanish-speaking managed care patient who occasionally has an Axis III orthopedic or neurological disorder, and who may seek help for the emotional aftermath of personal injury and disability.

Many Spanish-speaking immigrants also present in therapy with marital problems, as new roles and opportunities develop for women in the United States and as the more traditional Latino spouse may respond with anger or dismay to changing expectations. Also prevalent are disorders that affect children, particularly those who develop attention deficit disorders with hyperactivity. Parents become anxious over their own lack of expertise to make the school system responsive to their child's special needs, even though in many states they can personally request an individualized education plan for their offspring. Cases of anxiety, depression, and panic are no less frequent than with Anglo-American patients. These syndromes demand culturally relevant responses from the psychotherapist. Anger management is another area of need. Patients who are either mandated by the courts or themselves come for help are relatively frequent among men, women, and teenagers. Parent-child disputes and conflicts are another important area, and family therapy is necessary to help adolescents adjust to their parents' cultural expectations while they receive endless messages from the world at large to "do their own thing." Finally, sex therapy is an intervention that the psychotherapist may frequently find necessary, due to cultural factors that I will look at more closely.

PAIN CONTROL AND THE TREATMENT OF POST-TRAUMATIC STRESS DISORDER

The Spanish-speaking working poor who obtain managed care mental health coverage at their factories and work sites are often unskilled or semiskilled employees. They perform jobs that include repetitive and awkward movements as they lift, stretch, and stand many hours a day. This population does not commonly enter the managed care referral network for severe mental disorders, psychoses, delusions, or dissociative behaviors. By definition, the client is in the workforce and at least able to function at acceptable levels. Moreover, Latino patients are less likely to have sick leave, vacation time, or extended benefits. Thus, their schedules tend to be somewhat inflexible and attendance at psychotherapy is most likely to happen during evening hours after work, or in the morning before a second shift begins. If severe dysfunction occurs, it is the spouse or children who may be more likely to present with these problems. In addition to the personal and family issues presented by clients, they may frequently be under the care of a family physician or orthopedic specialist for their aches and pains. When this happens, many Latino immigrants harbor fears that they will not be able to continue working due to physical disability, especially given the excellent work ethic that characterizes this population. A gift of the hypnotic relaxation tape discussed in Chapter 3 can be very helpful to alleviate some of the client's symptoms. The tape can be further personalized using Hilgard and Hilgard's (1983) inductions for pain control, discussed next.

Generally, it is a good idea to write a scenario for the hypnosis tape with the patient at hand to alert him or her to the different techniques that will be included. Imagery of walking by the beach is not a good idea if that client almost drowned once while swimming in the ocean. Some of the techniques that I draw upon benefit from Hilgard and Hilgard's work on hypnosis and pain and include the following:

1. Imagine a small room with switches; you see yourself turning off the switches one by one, and each time, you feel more relief from discomfort. I use the poetic conceit that "just as you see yourself turning off the switches, so, too, do you keep any discomfort from coming to conscious awareness."

2. Imagine a green jar full of ice water. As you place your right hand in the jar, it becomes numb. Now, take your hand and massage the area of your body in need until the numbness passes to that area. Now, your right hand returns to normal and you feel very relaxed, calm, and tranquil.

3. After a short lecture on how neurons work and why they can send messages through the body laterally just as easily as linearly, I instruct the client as follows: Imagine yourself feeling any discomfort travel to the pinkie finger of your left hand, and from there, any discomfort now travels outward to the airwaves, leaving you feeling relaxed and calm.

4. Imagine that when you wake up early in the morning, you sit at the edge of your bed. For thirty seconds you will experience any discomfort connected to your condition; afterward, you are free of discomfort all day long.

5. Imagine yourself on a happy occasion (state the date of the birthday, Christmas, etc., of the year prior to the onset of the

injury) and that you feel as good now as you did on that eventful date.

If the client's pain results from trauma, hypnosis is very effective to alleviate the symptoms; moreover, trauma patients appear to be more responsive to hypnotic inductions than the public at large. It is very important that the client help design the tape. I use the first twenty minutes of a second session to personalize the tape, if necessary. This gift of healing is very dramatic, and patients return with high praise for their pain relief. Often, their depression and anxiety alleviate when they realize that they can effectively control their own body.

Exposure therapy works well with patients who have experienced a traumatic event that has propelled them into treatment. Clients are asked to repeat the details of the trauma during each session. To explain to them why they are so jittery and wound up, or hyper-aroused, I draw upon a particular story. I tell them that the nervous system is like an apartment with noisy neighbors upstairs. A trauma is an event like this, so when a neighbor drops one shoe, the body is tense, waiting for the second shoe to drop. We call this hyper-vigilance, and this explains why the traumatized person has trouble sleeping or relaxing. As the client repeats the details of the trauma again and again, relief is in store. In Spanish I tell clients that it is a paradox *(parece mentira),* but that the more they tell their stories "through their mouths," the less the stories will stay in their heads (with intrusive memories)—*mas que sale por la boca menos que queda en su cabeza!* The empowerment symbol of the eagle discussed in Chapter 2 is helpful in making the client feel in control. The client is instructed to listen to the tape twice daily and before going to sleep to dampen the hypervigilant state.

In my work on hypnosis and pain control (see de Rios and Friedman 1987), I noted that in shamanic techniques of healing, few questions are asked of the patient. The shaman is all-knowing and all-powerful and certain that the intervention will work. In my work with hypnosis, I find that metaphors are the best intervention possible. To ensure compliance with my instructions to listen to the hypnosis tape, and to reframe any lack of compliance, I use the metaphor of a child's seesaw. I tell clients that when the effects of the trauma are strong, they will need to listen to the tape often, but as they get better and more in control, just like the seesaw, they will need to use it less.

If clients are in physical or occupational therapy as part of their rehabilitation, additional segments can be added to the tape. I write a scenario with clients that describes the exercises to do both in the clinic and at home. Then, I reiterate on the tape that they feel calm and tranquil, and I use the symbol of the eagle to liken their endurance in the exercises to the strength and power of the mighty eagle, king of his dominion.

Latino Child Trauma: The Single-Blow Event

Spanish-speaking immigrant children frequently suffer single-event traumas, whether it be the ones I have seen at weekly burn rounds or those who have fallen off a ledge, been attacked by a dog, dragged by a bus, etc. Full-blown examples of post-traumatic stress disorder may ensue from these accidents. A particular type of play therapy that I call magical realism is effective and short term (de Rios 1997). It is a play therapy technique that is resonant with the child's cultural background and employs cultural symbols and beliefs. This is most useful when no death has occurred. I am particularly interested in the phenomenon of affective state-dependent retention and the memory trace for childhood trauma. The play therapy theory focuses on the traumatized child's hyperaroused states. I call upon cultural superheroes or heroines and villains during the play to help the child reexperience the trauma, but with a different outcome. The state of consciousness of the child remembering the trauma event means that there is an emotional arousal. The psychotherapist helps the child re-create the emotional state by the technique of mutual storytelling. However, in the psychotherapist's narrative, a superhero is called upon to vanquish the villain in the trauma. This enables the child to process the narrative memory of the event without the emotional intensity that accompanied the original experience. This catharsis restarts information processing, generates a less upsetting narrative memory of the traumatic event, and enables the child to master any anxiety that is provoked, which is detrimental to the developmental tasks that remain. Such an approach provides a culturally meaningful intervention to treat the psychological sequelae of the child's trauma. The following is a case study that illustrates how this technique operates.

The Case Study

Romero and Natalia were two Latino siblings, ages six and eight, with no prior psychological dysfunction or school problems. I received the referral for psychotherapy when the boy was run over by a small pickup truck the day before Halloween. The mother and two children were returning home from the store with costumes for trick or treat, when a truck turned the corner, ran over Romero, and caused his sister to fall. The mother witnessed the accident. Paramedics arrived shortly, and both children were kept overnight in a nearby hospital. Fortunately, Romero suffered only abrasions and no broken bones, although there was a fair amount of bleeding. The children were seen together in therapy twice a week for a four-month period. Although Romero and Natalia were in the first and third grades, respectively, they spoke Spanish at home. The family had migrated from a rural village in Mexico some five years earlier, and the father was employed as a laborer in construction. Both children developed a fear of crossing the street. Their mother, who had witnessed the accident, developed tachycardia, and I treated her separately.

The intervention consisted of play therapy so that the children could reenact the trauma. I used a toy truck as a prop and placed in the truck bed an ugly doll of bright primary colors, with one foot ending in a tail, rolling eyes, and a moveable jaw—in short, a monster doll. Appropriate mestizo dolls were used to represent the mother and children. Additionally, nurse and doctor dolls, a toy ambulance, and a hospital bedroom scene were used in the reenactment. I modified Gardner's (1971) mutual storytelling technique. The children were instructed first to enact the trauma scene for my benefit. I encouraged them to tell the story as loudly and dramatically as they could. After the children told the story, it was my turn to reenact it. In this second telling, I introduced a superhero/religious figure, namely a statue of Jesus, which I used to knock the monster out of the truck. I threw the monster against the wall with a loud noise and lots of enthusiasm. Then I made a "magical circle" around the children with the statue of Jesus, which I said would protect them whenever they crossed the street. Interestingly, the children never considered that Jesus had failed them in any way by not preventing the accident from occurring in the first place, although one could say he prevented them from being seriously injured.

During each session, I asked the children to draw whatever they wished. When prompted, they drew scenes of the traumatic event. Over a period of ten sessions, I obtained crayon drawings that painstakingly re-created the details of the accident. Subsequently, the children became bored with the activity and began to draw other scenes of animals, birds, butterflies, houses, etc. I discharged them from therapy at this point, as the trauma had become very routinized. They reenacted the accident and resolved their anxiety with the help of a religious statue of Jesus, which was an important symbol for them and their family. At a follow-up inquiry one year later, the children were reported to be doing fine, making good progress in their schoolwork, and with no reports of bad dreams, re-enactments of the trauma, or behavioral problems.

The introduction of Jesus as a protective figure allowed both children to explore and become desensitized as well as to create a more favorable outcome through play. What the protective image of Jesus may have accomplished was to provide a sufficient sense of emotional support or safety, a "testimonial witness," so that the children were able to overcome the fears that prohibited independent learning of the rules of street safety. Such a traumatized child might neither cross the street nor look both ways without arousing intolerable fear. The choice of the Jesus image was culturally acceptable as well as resonant with the beliefs and values of the community and the family. I suppose any other powerful figure, regardless of its cultural meaning, could have been utilized in the intervention. Anthropologists, however, who argue that our cultural membership conditions who we define as powerful and significant figures, would agree that attention should be paid to particularistic rather than universal kinds of features, e.g., a legendary or mythic figure as opposed to a tiger or lion as a symbol of strength.

MARITAL PROBLEMS AMONG IMMIGRANTS

Some interesting patterns are beginning to emerge with regard to gender issues and migration. The psychotherapist has to pay attention to relationships between men and women as the result of immigration, especially with regard to the immigrants' area of origin and their socioeconomic background. Important factors include whether a man emigrated from a small hamlet, where he was obliged to support his wife and children. Is the wife typically the homemaker, or, at best, a peddler selling food from a cart? Or does the client come from an outlying slum in north Mexico City, where men, women, and children are busy at work in commercial activities, selling goods in order to make ends meet? Or is the wife the daughter of a small government bureaucrat, who was expected to stay home and embroider, work around the house and wait for a husband to take her off her father's hands? Women have many different expectations with regard to their role in life. Immigration simply magnifies expectations. For example, when Blanca and Eduardo fell in love, they never gave social class differences a thought. Like some soap opera on Spanish-language TV when an Indian girl loves and marries an industrial tycoon, Blanca and Eduardo came from different social categories in Mexico. Eduardo had clawed his way out of a dysfunctional family, became a school teacher, and had sufficient economic resources. His excessive jealousy and need to control the movements of his wife, who came from a loving, middle-class background, caused a rupture, and there were hints of potential domestic violence directed against Blanca. At the end of five visits, she left home and moved in with her older sister and brother-in-law.

Many Latino couples stay together over the years, despite bad marriages and unhealthy squabbling. Marilu finally left her husband on her sixty-fifth birthday, as she could not stand his petty ways and vindictive behavior any longer. She lived on her Social Security income and was adamant in my office that her ex-husband was cheating her by not sharing income that he received from rental property that they jointly held. Far too often, women socialized in Mexico in childhood and adolescence leave business matters in their husbands' hands. Some, such as Marilu, learn in the school of hard knocks when their husbands keep resources hidden from them or actually cheat on them. Generally, they are cash poor and unable to pay a lawyer to help them rectify the problem.

A large number of Spanish-speaking clients in managed care are couples in which both spouses work, even though gender expectations from Latin America may not have changed very much. Many women are angry that they have to work in dead-end jobs that are both dangerous and fatiguing. When Spanish-speaking married women find their way into the worker's compensation system after a burn or orthopedic injury, they often express strong anger against their husbands, whose idea it often was for them to take that job in the first place.

Other women typically enjoy receiving a paycheck, as well as the buying power and independence that such work bestows. Among most of the Latino couples whom I have counseled, the women often commingle their money with that of their husbands. On some occasions, when a marriage is going badly and separation looms on the horizon, a housewife will complain that she dare not seek a job because her husband will simply stop giving her money for food and rent.

When the issue is battering or verbal abuse of the wife and family, or alcoholism, the psychotherapist must evaluate the the kind of social network available to the woman to ensure that she can be protected from continued beatings or abuse. Too often, parents and adult brothers or sisters remain in Latin America and may not be able to help out if there are also severe economic problems. Remittances flow from the United States to other countries, not vice-versa. It is important to explain to clients about the U.S. criminal justice system and how essential it is for the wife to create a paper trail to document the husband's misbehavior if any beatings are involved. Clients almost always know about 911 service, but the psychotherapist has to make it clear that the wife must inform her husband that beatings will not be tolerated. I find it is very helpful as I sit with the client to pull out of my bookcase one of the excellent psychotherapy volumes available concerning the battered woman syndrome. I translate freely so that the client is able to see her own sorry pattern coincide with the words of "experts." This often brings tears to her eyes, as many a battered woman deludes herself that this cycle of battering and romantic reconciliations will end and that a normal relationship will finally ensue. I try to arrange for the husband to come into therapy, but often this is not successful. Many batterers desire to control their wives and their movements. This includes keeping a woman out of contact with others who could loosen the control the man may have over her. In Latino culture, men who batter typically hold traditional hierarchical beliefs, are emotionally inexpressive, have low self-esteem, use violence to achieve superiority, and have vocational problems (see Casas et al. 1994).

The use of experts to explicate a problem is an analogic technique that I learned from the shamanic healers whom I studied in Peru. Known as a *vidente* (seer; see de Rios 1984b), the healer uses either well-developed intuition or "second sight" to bring forth secrets and hidden information about the client's personal life. In my case, I choose to employ a well-argued and reasoned sociological discussion about the battered wife syndrome which conveys the idea that the psychotherapist, too, is a *vidente*, able to uncover those terrible secrets and bring them to light. I have watched clients experience abreaction and catharsis as the result of this technique. This has led to the next step of persuading the husband to come in for treatment or else for the wife to consider separation.

Alina and her husband were a good example of this. In the first session, Alina spoke in general terms of her marital problems with Edgar. On the second session, however, she was tearful and black and blue with a swollen cheek. She slowly revealed information about the events leading to Edgar beating her. Alina responded dramatically to the sociological pattern of battering that I discussed with her from one of my reference books. At the next session, her husband accompanied her and we were able to develop specific cognitive techniques to help him correct his distorted thinking processes about his need to control his wife's movements. At such times, I draw further analogies as I point to the conference room next door where I hold anger management classes each week. I indicated to Edgar that there, but for the grace of God, he might have to go each week and that if he continued to beat Alina, he and his wife ran the risk of having their children taken from the home, should authorities view it as a dangerous place for the youngsters. Unlike typical bibliotherapy, in which the client is sent home to read an authoritative volume, the psychotherapist must bridge the world of research to that of the client and apply relevant findings to help the client understand the causes and possible resolution for the clinical issues.

Needless to say, a psychotherapist must be able to inform the client how to obtain a restraining order and should have at hand a regional telephone number for a domestic violence unit where Spanish is spoken. Names and telephone numbers of women's shelters are also important to keep within easy reach. It is not unusual in Southern California, for example, to find a sizable Spanish-speaking population in residence in any shelter at any given time. The psychotherapist, too, should keep a file on ESL (English as a second language) to enhance the client's employability, as well as inexpensive resources for baby-sitting, addresses of boys' and girls' clubs, etc. Many Latina immigrants come from families where they may have seen their mother abused by a violent drunken father. These women are discouraged from earliest youth from being assertive or independent and are taught to be passive and compliant. They frequently become depressed and present with issues of low self-esteem. As acculturation pressures influence immigrant women and allow them to see other options, they are less likely to *aguantar*—suffer in silence or remain immobilized.

Maria Elena, a beautiful young woman of twenty-eight, was entranced by her boyfriend, a sadistic, insulting man who kept her off-balance with his manipulative behavior. By learning assertiveness training, she was able to confront him and stand up for her rights. As it turned out, Maria Elena's sense of self-worth improved considerably when she passed her real estate licensing examination after diligent study. As with many other people, she realized that no one could take away from her whatever she achieved educationally, which literally came from the sweat of her brow. A hypnosis tape in Spanish designed to enhance her ability to remember studied materials and to control her test-taking anxiety helped her to relax and stay focused.

Not all low self-esteem clients are easy to treat. Marta's husband had a *casa chica* or other household in Mexico, and he was spending vacations and other free time with his girlfriend. One of the effects of acculturation on Marta was to boost her own sense of self and to persuade her to go it alone without the husband. Even with only minimal education, she could scratch out a living for herself and her children and get by without the humiliation of being a concubine. Marta might not have known what the word "feminism" meant, but she understood the principle of equal rights and the sanctity of the household.

A pattern that I see among couples who have managed care insurance occurs when a Mexican-American woman, born and educated in the United States, marries a young Mexican or Latin American immigrant with little education or skills. Typically the man becomes very dependent upon his wife, who is in charge of paying bills and obtaining loans, credit cards, a home mortgage, etc. This gives her a certain leverage in the relationship, which translates into her demands for equal treatment and rights. Men with traditional Mexican or South American backgrounds, however, often become angry in these relationships, feel inadequate, and suffer from anxiety. They may turn to alcohol and nights out with their friends to assert their independence and to reestablish a marital pattern closer to their expectations of marriage back in Mexico or Latin America. Both Latina women born in the States and those who are immigrants develop less tolerance for the independent husband who hangs out with his buddies and drinks away his wages. The more acculturated the immigrant woman becomes, the less likely she is to permit this to continue without considering separation or divorce. Nonetheless, such women often worry about their children being left homeless or without a father, and many reflect upon their own upbringing and any similar circumstances in their own personal history.

Latina immigrant women often must learn techniques of assertiveness that were not available to them in their families of origin in Latin America. Appendix B includes a chart I prepared in Spanish and English as a psychoeducational technique to help women clients learn nonaggressive ways to try to get their needs met. I role-play with women if they need to try out the technique, which is often quite a new experience for them. In contrast to a direct technique such as this, many women have perfected indirect manipulation, and a direct, frontal approach is not easy for them. However, manipulation does appear to meet many of their needs. The indirect technique works very well in third world cultures where male dominance is the norm.

As a graduate student I had occasion to conduct archaeological research as part of a university group in a small Anatolian village in Turkey. One late afternoon, as our student group was taking a walk around the village of 300 people, we turned a corner and saw about fifty women lounging in the shade of a tree, in deep conversation. Always the anthropologist, I inquired of our seventeen-year-old male interpreter from a local city high school, who was spending the summer helping to interpret for the group. The young man, with a sheepish grin on his face, replied that the women were discussing the sexual inadequacies of their husbands! This in an area of the world where men were commonly rough and physically abusive in their treatment of their wives. Thus, the oppressed women can use mockery as a tool to make their husbands treat them reasonably.

ATTENTION DEFICIT DISORDERS
WITH HYPERACTIVITY

Nationally, it is estimated that one in six children in the United States suffers from attention deficit disorder with hyperactivity. Since the working poor have little money for preschools for their children and often leave their youngsters in the care of relatives, three-, four-, and five-year-old children who suffer this disorder often are not evaluated by professionals until they enter kindergarten or first grade. For the family involved, however, these children can be a real problem and cause them a good deal of concern. Once a managed care contract is in hand, the Latino family rarely hesitates to bring in such a child for counseling.

For purposes of assessment, I have found that the Hawthorne Scales in Spanish are very useful (McCarney, 1994). The psychotherapist can sit with either or both parents to determine if the child merits a diagnosis of ADHD. Although managed care companies generally do not authorize testing, the scales only take about ten to fifteen minutes to administer, and since the psychotherapist is interactive with the parents, a case can be made that this, in itself, is a therapeutic experience. Once analyzed (taking up another few minutes at most), the psychotherapist can call or write the child's pediatrician or family doctor to discuss results and request a medication evaluation. McCarney and Bauer's (1994) volume that accompanies the scales can be kept handy in the office. For each area of concern—inattention, impulsivity, and hyperactivity—there are very straightforward and direct instructions (in English, unfortunately), for detailed behavior modification techniques that family members can utilize on a daily basis to ensure that the child learns to control these traits.

In many cases, the scales enable the psychotherapist to rule out ADHD and in its place to uncover power struggles between the parents, who use the child as a scapegoat or designated patient. David is a good example of this. A bright seven-year-old, David was brought in by his bickering parents due to his difficulties in school, particularly with learning the alphabet and acquiring writing skills. What emerged was that the child had a learning disability, although his father was so angry at his wife that he refused to seek help for the child and only accompanied the family to therapy because of his wife's nagging. Fortunately, the school was willing to test the child and provide the necessary resources to deal with his learning problem. As might be expected, this youngster was able to play one parent against the other, which added to the delay to diagnose and treat his problem.

Another clinical issue that mirrors ADHD is the treatment of the child who is *consentido,* or excessively spoiled by the parents. Such a child often misbehaves, and teachers are not likely to tolerate misbehavior in their classrooms as do the child's parents at home. Sometimes hyperactivity, inattention, or impulsivity traits may be reported by the teacher. Dulcina was a fifty-one-year-old mother of a nine-year-old child, Ruben, who was disruptive in school. After evaluating the child and interviewing the mother, it was clear to me that Ruben was an only child, born late in her life, and the mother could not find it in her heart to discipline him.

In these cases of spoiled children, I generally use the metaphor of criminality when I speak to mothers. I talk about what the child is really learning when he always gets his way. Is it that life exists solely to please him? When he grows up, he will not always get what he wants and will, in some cases, take what he needs. The outcome we can expect may include a criminal career. Most parents immediately think of neighborhood gang violence, drug dealing, etc., and get the message about the need to set limits for their children. Providing a workbook on behavior modification for sale (the STEP program in Spanish) and some discussion of the principles involved is the next step. Next to my psychotherapy couch, I have a framed snapshot that I took in an aquarium of a 3,000 pound killer whale who is jumping straight in the air (a lucky shot!). I tell the parent about the principle of how trainers reward random movements of this huge mammal by giving it gifts of small fish. If a trainer can make a huge whale who weighs more than my car jump that high, it will be easy for the parent to modify the child's behavior.

One of the roles of the psychotherapist in the case of ADHD and other learning disorders that children may suffer is to be a voice for the family, a *vocera*—to bring to the school's attention the child's need for smaller classes, personalized teaching, special education resources, individualized educational plans, etc. Often, when the psychotherapist makes a formal request for school records on business stationery, the school gets the message that someone with psychological credentials is paying attention. At that juncture, a school psychologist may suddenly appear out of nowhere, at least to test the child within ninety days, at most. The child probably has been in need of evaluation for a long time. Knowing the name of a good lawyer or two who specialize in children's rights is also useful leverage to combat any institutional racism that may be either latent or rampant in a particular school district.

One should also have on hand the names of Spanish-speaking psychologists who specialize in neuropsychological testing at reasonable rates. If there is a major problem with a child's educability, I recommend a consultation, testing, and evaluation letter from such a psychologist, which unfortunately the parents must often pay for out of pocket. There is also a state-funded developmental disability agency in our area that provides services in Spanish. I keep their advertisements on hand as another referral source for needy clients.

One must be optimistic with these clients, even when a child appears to be mildly mentally retarded, as it is important to give the parents hope for the future. A graduate student of mine wrote her master's thesis on mentally retarded children in Mexico and their parents' perceptions of their children's problems (Schoef, 1995). In a significant number of cases, parents there did not want to accept the finality of the diagnosis of retardation and were certain that their children would be able to learn a trade and make a living as adults. This may be more possible in an agrarian, developing society such as Mexico or other parts of Latin America where opportunities for manual labor are very common. In Southern California, following the NAFTA agreement, numerous factories relocated to Mexico and Asia, and unskilled laborers are now less likely to find work.

Last, but not least, it is important to check out the child's diet and nutrition, even if the psychotherapist is not particularly cognizant of the finer points of biochemistry. In third world countries, fresh produce is trucked daily to markets and is purchased each day. Moreover, each meal is prepared from scratch, not made from boxed ingredients with food coloring, additives, fructose, MSG, or artificial flavorings. Given the fast pace of everyday life, immigrant mothers, as with everyone else, have less time to prepare nutritious meals for their families. Miguel, a five-year-old boy, came to see me with his parents because not only was he hyperactive but also he woke up with nightmares and saw green monsters in the closet, which he obligingly drew for me. Scanning a list of his typical meals that I elicited from his parents, I realized that he was drinking preparations that were chemical banquets, with additives galore. I asked the parents to modify his diet with fruit juices and to introduce more fruits and vegetables into his daily intake. We scheduled the next appointment for two weeks down the line. When the family arrived (and sheepishly I may add), the problem had mostly disappeared. The poor child's liver apparently could not tolerate his fast-food intake. If only all cases were so easy to treat!

ANXIETY AND DEPRESSION

Men and women come to counseling because of depression and *los nervios* (nerves). Writers such as Vega and colleagues (1991) suggest that as a result of immigration, Mexican immigrants have smaller interaction networks than subsequent generations and are more likely to rely on family for emotional support. Many immigrants experience a loss when they leave their homeland and sever personal ties that give meaning and significance to their lives. Vega, Kolody, and Valle (1987) found that some immigrants express this loss through depressive symptoms. If social resources are available in the receiving environment of the immigrant, this will contribute to satisfactory adaptation, including the avoidance of mental health problems that are associated with disrupted social support networks. Often, it takes a certain period of time before social networks are reconstituted, which has implications for emotional support.

Vega's research in San Diego with an immigrant group (Vega et al., 1991) shows that at least 81 percent of respondents had annual contact with a brother or sister and more than half with a parent. Only about 10 percent of his sample had little or no contact with the family of origin. Those women who lacked employment, who had a low educational level, and who did not drive a car, in turn, had fewer social contacts and less perceived support, which correlated with higher depression. Vega found that immigrants do use social networks as a primary resource and are active in these networks to acquire the basic requirements for survival. It may be that immigrants are not necessarily at greater risk for mental illness when they are able to utilize social resources available to them. His findings suggest that Mexican immigrant women who have had to sever their social networks in Mexico are readily able to join or create new ones in the United States. These comprise both friends and family contacts, which persist over time.

Dissociative behavior is much more rare than depression and is more frequently reported among Cuban and Puerto Rican clients in the psychotherapy literature. In Southern California, the typical client is of Mexican origin, with fewer originating from Central and South America. Afro-Cuban influences in the Caribbean do correlate with dissociative behaviors more frequently than elsewhere, and they have a cultural value and influence. Occasionally, clients will come into treatment while they are taking medicines they purchased from a *botanica,* or herbal shop, and many go back and forth to the border city of Tijuana, Mexico, to purchase medicines not legally available in the United States without a prescription.

Causes of depression are multiple among this community of immigrants. Many suffer from economic stress. I am always amazed at the large number of clients I see who have mortgages *hasta las nubes,* up in the clouds, that is, $1,400 - $1,800 per month, with a couple's salaries probably not exceeding $35,000 per year, and often less. There are any number of unscrupulous mortgage brokers in the region who prey on the community and falsify clients' tax documents to permit individuals with moderate incomes to purchase houses that are simply far beyond their means. The dream of having your own home is fine, but it can become a nightmare when the mortgage is out of sight and job security is uncertain. Many report losing their homes and whatever equity they were able to save for a down payment. Others experience nostalgia for their homeland. This is not an uncommon complaint, despite the fact that many areas of the region where they now live have Spanish-language shopping, movies, swap meets, etc. Some women suffer postpartum depression in mild or moderate form and are constantly tired from taking care of an infant, attending to the needs of other children in the household, and waiting on their husbands, who may do precious few chores around the house.

As mentioned in Chapter 4, it is important to assess very early on if the client will benefit from psychiatric medication. If so, the psychotherapist must make the referral as quickly as possible. I employ a metaphor about how the brain works and why medication can be good for the client. Many people are fearful that such medications will make them crazy *(loco)* if they have to take a pill every day in order to feel good. The metaphor that I use is one of malabsorption, which compares psychiatric medication to the problems facing diabetics, a condition not uncommon in the Latino community. The argument goes as follows: just as insulin allows the diabetic to absorb sugar, so too does the SSRI (selective serotonin reuptake inhibitor) medication help the client to absorb his or her own serotonin. People feel better after viewing the little drawings that I make for them to show how the medication is an intermediary to enable them to absorb their own brain chemicals so that they do not experience distress. I often ask the spouse to be present when I draw this diagram, so that he or she will encourage the client to continue taking the medication. Figure 6.1 shows the chart that I draw to show my clients what a neuron looks like. The dialogue that accompanies it follows.

> Many of the cells in your body are like A, B, C, and D in this drawing. You see that they share a wall together, much like a fence between neighbors' properties. When you walk or run a lot, you perspire and the salt goes out of A. He borrows some from B over the fence, and you know that is happening because you may get a cramp in your leg, since cell B no longer has enough of its own salt. Now, the cells in your brain, spinal cord, and nerves are different because they do not share a cell wall.
>
> If A and B in Figure 6.1 want to communicate, cell A has to make a chemical and zap it electrically to B (it's as though A is upriver and B is downriver). Then, along comes C. He is like the cartoon figure, Popeye, with his mop, and since these chemicals are like liquids, Popeye has to mop up any spill. Then C goes over to D, who is like this thermostat in my office, and C tells him to make more or less of the chemical. Now sometimes,

FIGURE 6.1. Neurons and the Effects of Antidepressant Medication on Them

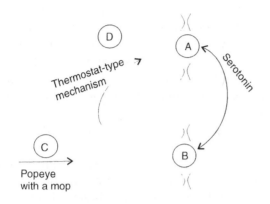

Close-up of cell B after antidepressant medication first started:

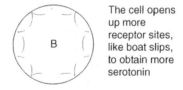

The cell opens up more receptor sites, like boat slips, to obtain more serotonin

Why You Should Take Psychiatric Medication

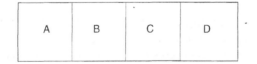

because you inherited the condition or because of the stress *(la carga emocional)* that you are currently experiencing, this delicate mechanism doesn't work so well. Popeye in fact is working overtime to mop up your own brain chemical, serotonin, before it can be absorbed into your body, into B. So, let's look at the medicine that the doctor may want you to take. It is called an

SSRI. S means to select; the other S is serotonin, which affects your mood; the R is reuptake like a sponge; and I is inhibiting or preventing the chemical from getting into your cell. [Then I explain by drawing an insert of cell B.] Once you start the psychiatric medication, cell B is so happy to get its own chemical that it opens up boat slips *(muelles)* or docks for the first few days or weeks to suck up the medication. This may account for some mild discomfort, but once you get back on track, B closes down the extra docks and the cell returns to normal.

With regard to issues of anxiety, the relaxation tape is very helpful. The empowerment image of the eagle helps the client to feel in control again. The psychotherapist must be a practical person with common sense to help resolve clients' basic problems of living in the areas of economic, legal, and vocational issues. In an employee assistance program supervisor-generated referral that authorized just one visit, the tardiness and emotional stress of the Spanish-speaking client was exacerbated by the fact that she lived fifty-five miles from the factory (which had relocated from her home community to a more distant one). Her car was old and worn, and broke down frequently. My advice: "Get another job, young lady, or move closer." This may seem trite, but it apparently was some kind of revelation to the client.

ANGER MANAGEMENT

Young Latino immigrants often find themselves enmeshed in the criminal justice system if they are unable to control their anger, as they become involved in physical or verbal altercations with spouses, girlfriends, or outsiders, or if they have an attitude problem with police officers. Women may become violent over a love affair gone sour, betrayal by a boyfriend or lover, or as the result of verbal abuse. Isabel's experience was not atypical. She had been living with Silvestre for ten years when her daughter from a former marriage, who suffered from the sleep disorder of somnambulence, got into bed with her and her husband one night. The husband, who later claimed that he was asleep, assumed that his wife was caressing him, and he began to make love to the child. Isabel woke up, screamed, and got the child back to her own bed. Her daughter had no memory of the event. The couple separated, as Isabel moved out with her three children. Some two months later, without success in reconciling, Isabel showed up unannounced at her old apartment and found Silvestre in bed with a woman lodger. Unable to contain her anger, she began to cut up old photographs, break crockery, and generally lose control. When the police arrived, Silvestre exaggerated the events and told the police that his wife had tried to kill him. The couple eventually reunited and used their seven sessions for marital counseling to learn cognitive techniques to solve problems and to enhance their communication skills. One of my functions in this case was to prepare a succinct report for the court, in this case, to help reduce Isabel's possible three-month jail sentence to fifteen days.

I provide several classes in Spanish for both men and women who have had altercations with others. The program focuses on nondomestic violence and serves individuals who have been mandated by the courts for ten weeks of training to learn to control their anger. Additionally, clients with managed care coverage also seek help for similar problems, although the sessions available to them are frequently fewer in number.

Dr. Weisinger's Anger Work-Out Book (Weisinger, 1985) is a helpful volume to use in this training, although it is not available in Spanish. I provide a running translation of one or more chapters for each class. The book basically helps the client understand the physiology of anger, as well as helping him or her develop a number of cognitive techniques to control angry thoughts, to keep body chemistry in control, and to minimize negative events that would lead to future altercations with others. Since the anger management classes that are mandated by the courts have to be paid for by the client, people prefer to access these services through their mental health insurance when available and then request a brief letter from the psychotherapist at the conclusion of training to indicate that anger issues have been addressed successfully. In effect, it is easier to work with this population through managed care than through court mandates. For example, if the client should be diagnosed with a bipolar disorder, as often happens, the psychotherapist can recommend a medication evaluation, which is much more difficult to set up for a self-paying court-mandated client. Such clients generally have sufficient trouble finding resources to pay the small fee for group therapy, let alone the cost of psychiatric medication or a doctor's fee if the client does not have insurance. Once they are prescribed psychiatric medication, many individuals will go to a Mexican border town to purchase their medicine at half the out-of-pocket costs they would have to pay in California.

When the psychotherapist provides group therapy for anger management, other brief interventions with these clients may develop, since angry people typically have a host of problems to deal with. These may include dysthymia from the economic setbacks they have to endure to pay their fines and to make restitution for any damage to the victim's property or hospital bills. Many clients are quite bitter about their experiences with the law and have the potential to become antisocial if their anger is not diffused and if they are unable or unwilling to take responsibility for their own acts. In men's groups, one typically finds a self-styled leader who is quick to get up on a soapbox and air his gripes while others who may be more closed-mouthed remain in the background. The psychotherapist has to work hard to call upon each and every client to illustrate the point being discussed. Metaphor is useful here to make certain points clear. Most of the Latino clients, to date, with whom I have worked have less than a high school education. Male immigrants often do not have much of an idea of how the U.S. legal system works, what the rules are, and how they are enforced. I am offered bribes (unsolicited and unaccepted, I may add) at least twice a month from clients who request a certificate of completion for the courts. They hope that they will not have to attend any sessions. I gently explain that that is not how things are done here. If the client would benefit from it, I usually recommend a book in both languages, *The Law and Your Rights* (Araujo, 1998; see Appendix B), which is informative on contract and criminal law.

When I lived in Mexico and South America, I learned that part of the cost of doing business was the gratuities or bribes that were handed out to make bureaucrats responsive to the needs of their public. In the United States, when bribes are offered for such fraudulent purposes as those just mentioned, the psychotherapist has to be careful not to take personal offense, since the event may have an impersonal quality and culturally be expected. If anything, one could argue that by offering a bribe, the client shows trust that you will not make a problem for him or her if you decide not to accept. Most of my anger management group participants are aware that you cannot offer a bribe to a U.S. police officer, as you would surely do in Mexico or other parts of Latin America.

PANIC DISORDERS

Both men and women come to therapy suffering from panic disorders, often with few precipitating stressors. I do not see many phobic disorders, such as fear of heights, closed spaces, or flying. The onset of panic is often sudden. Laura is a good example. She never had any kind of panic attack until she went back home to Mexico after three years in the United States, despite the fact that she had no documents to enable her to cross the border again. Most of her vacation was ruined as all she could think about was how she would return. She had a very dangerous crossing and was apprehended by the border patrol. She was returned to Mexico before she could cross again. Although she now has legal documents, she developed agoraphobia as a response to her trauma, and she often thinks she is going to have a heart attack.

Medical evaluations for these patients are essential, and antianxiety medications such as Buspar and Wellbutrin are very important in panic control. I teach the client deep breathing techniques and some yoga techniques of nasal breathing. When an individual needs to quiet his or her mind, I bring out some meditative mantras from the 1960s and teach the client to repeat the phrase, "Om shakti, Om shakti, Om shakti, Om" (for a ten-minute period). These techniques of quieting the mind help to minimize intrusive thoughts that can be very upsetting to the client. I draw a diagram to explain brain waves and states of consciousness. I focus on four major states: deep sleep, dreaming, relaxation, and concentration (see Figure 6.2). I use the following dialogue to describe the diagram.

You know, there is a field of psychology that studies what goes on electrically in your brain, which is called biofeedback. The way it works is simple. Imagine a machine with three electrodes that I would paste on your forehead. This picks up

FIGURE 6.2. States of Consciousness

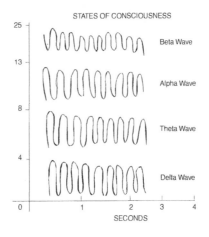

electrical activity inside your head. Then the machine magnifies it (like amplification in your stereo set). Then this electricity is converted into an electrical current that moves a pen across a piece of paper, as in the diagram (Figure 6.2). Sometimes the brain wave patterns are random, although many times they are entrained or fall into a particular pattern.

First, we have the delta wave, which is that of deep sleep. Then we have the theta wave, which is what happens when you are dreaming. Then we have the alpha wave, which is deep relaxation, important for your body to self-regulate and to monitor all the hormones and secretions. You know, your body is like a chemical factory. Then we have beta waves, which are for concentration and problem solving. If you wake up while you are in delta sleep, you may need to have a strong cup of coffee to become alert. If you are balancing your checkbook late at night, you may have problems getting your brain electricity low enough to fall asleep quickly.

If clients are hyperalert and agitated, I suggest that they probably are producing beta waves. I illustrate our goal of getting the clients to sleep well and to relax by references to the diagram and how important it is for them to learn to produce alpha waves. This technique is also very helpful in teaching pain patients how to distance themselves from their pain. The relaxation tape that I provide is an essential first step in treating both agitated and pain patients. I also use the first two therapy hours to provide direct hypnosis training for panic patients, to show them how much immediate relief they can obtain by listening to the tape and effectively, become relaxation virtuosos. A cognitive evaluation of clients' irrational beliefs also must be done quickly. In each of the following two or three sessions, I rhetorically challenge these beliefs and try to help clients realize that their expectations of the world they live in are excessive. Once these irrational beliefs become clear, I may resume hypnosis training and use systematic desensitization techniques to re-create in clients' minds a scene that has caused them to panic. I use hypnotic relaxation techniques at each stage of the desensitization, so that clients basically learn to quiet themselves. It takes about seven or eight sessions to provide relief for panic patients. Considering the frequency of their hospital visits when clients fears that they will die of a heart attack, the cost factor to the insurer can be considerably reduced. One medical group that I know actually proposed maintaining a salaried driver and van to pick up panic patients at their homes and shuttle them to the psychotherapy clinic to cut down managed care costs of emergency room evaluations for heart attacks!

SEXUAL DYSFUNCTION

As the result of my anthropological research in the Amazon, I became very interested in learning about hunting and gathering societies. It was not until the advent of agriculture that families began to have large numbers of children. By contrast, in hunting and gathering societies, women typically had about five offspring, not the ten to fourteen children that we see more commonly among rural and urban Latin American people. Without the safety net of a social security system for the elderly in most Central and South American countries, it is an advantage to have many children to secure one's old age.

Many of the immigrants I treat in managed care who suffer from sexual dysfunction were born into large families. They are often middle children and frequently report mild neglect in childhood. The phrase *"A que me sirve este hijo?"* (What use is this particular child to me?) is not uncommon to hear from women with numerous children. Such children are often scapegoated for one reason or another. They receive few hugs or caresses from their mothers. As babies they are held infrequently, as mother's duties in the household are overwhelming. Such children are subject to the cruel ministrations of older siblings—the ubiquitous child nurse so familiar in Latin American society. It is not surprising that when these men and women mature, they are not very sensual in their lovemaking and show little affection and gentleness, in turn, toward their mates. Mix this with a depression or anxiety disorder and oftentimes their marriages falter.

Juliano exemplified this process. He insists that his mother had nineteen children in Mexico, only ten of whom survived in extreme poverty conditions. A middle child, Juliano had little of his mother's attention. As an adult, Juliano was a womanizer whose constant sexual encounters troubled both his wives, who eventually left him. In his case, excessive sexual behavior was compensatory for the touch and attention he lacked as a child.

The psychotherapist must be alert to the possibility that many clients will need to be evaluated for sexual dysfunction. The therapist must be proactive in requesting information about the client's intimate life. Over the years as I have worked with Spanish-speaking burn patients, I realized that if I did not ask about sexual function, couples might go one and a half to two years without having sexual intercourse because of problems related to self-esteem, disfigurement issues, etc. Let's look at two cases.

A forty-five-year-old Mexican factory worker, Mr. Juarez suffered full-thickness burns to his right leg when he slipped while cleaning a vat, immersing his leg in a tub of chemicals. He underwent a skin graft procedure. The patient was depressed and anxious and had frequent flashbacks of the accident. He also had problems sleeping. The physician prescribed a tricyclic antidepressant, which Mr. Juarez took for a three-month period. Two years after his burns, while he was still being treated for pain in the donor site, he told me that he and his wife had abstained from sexual intercourse for these past two years. I began sexual therapy for the patient and his wife, and they resumed normal sexual relations with no problems reported. I taught them to do home exercises, which consisted of sensate focusing techniques as described by Singer (1974) to desensitize the client to premature ejaculation, which often follows traumatic injury. The client did not suffer from this problem before his accident.

A forty-one-year-old Cuban woman, Esmeralda, suffered burns to 30 percent of her body when the catering truck in which she worked as a cook collided with another vehicle and hot coffee spilled all over her. They were mostly second- and third-degree burns to her back, buttocks, and the back of her thighs. She was prescribed an anti-depressant medication for her depression, anxiety, and sleep disturbances, and she experienced sexual arousal dysfunction. This resulted in a reduced frequency of sexual intercourse with her husband. The medication was discontinued after several months as her trauma response lessened and she reported more frequent sexual intercourse. However, she experienced low self-esteem in the wake of disfigurement of her inner thigh and buttocks area.

As this case shows, when clients are depressed or suffer from trauma, they often lose interest in sex. Latino immigrants are quick to accuse the traumatized spouse of having an affair and of being unfaithful. They may be jealous of the spouse's movements and activities. The psychotherapist needs to explain to the couple about post-traumatic stress disorder to minimize these nonadaptive responses. Often SSRI medications are indicated, which in themselves can create additional problems for the client if they suppress sexual arousal. Benzodiazepines and antidepressants have become the standard of care not only with trauma patients but in general. A large body of literature has emerged on the sexual side effects of antidepressant medications.

My colleague Dr. Andrei Novac has written about how psychotropics may alter sex functions by a variety of mechanisms, including central nervous system (CNS) effects (sedation), CNS neurotransmitter effects (e.g., antidopaminergic effects on the hypothalamus), different peripheral neurotransmitter effects (e.g., alpha-adrenergic effects, which may interfere with erection), and hormonal effects (e.g., increase in prolactin caused by dopamine-blocking agents). Medications such as tricyclic antidepressants with their anticholinergic side effects often interfere with the cholinergic mechanisms that control erection and the adrenergically mediated emission phase of orgasm. Likewise, SSRIs such as fluoxetine hydrochloride, sertraline hydrochloride, and paroxetine hydrochloride are all known to interfere with libido, erection, and orgasm. A study conducted by Balon and colleagues (1993) found an overall incidence of sexual dysfunction of 45 percent among patients treated with antidepressants. These included decreased libido, difficulty reaching orgasm, painful orgasm (in men), and erectile dysfunction. Although such medications have been found to provide a valuable tool in psychiatric treatment, the potential for iatrogenically induced sexual dysfunction has to be recognized and treated when necessary. This may entail a change of medication, a lowered dosage, or simply informing the patient of the cost-benefit ratio to enable him or her to make an informed decision.

PSYCHOPHARMACOLOGY AND THE SPANISH-SPEAKING PATIENT

A growing scientific literature exists that examines ethnicity as an important factor to determine the response of patients to a wide variety of medications, including psychiatric ones, which are of major clinical significance to the psychotherapist. Much of this discussion draws on the work of Lin, Poland, and Anderson (1995) at the Harbor/UCLA Medical Center. From an evolutionary perspective, it makes good sense that any pharmacogenetic variability both between and within ethnic groups would have helped to ensure the survival of a population and a species that has to deal with toxic chemicals in its milieu.

Lin, a psychiatrist, has been conducting research for a number of years with colleagues to rectify the bias and lopsidedness of drug development research in the past, as a majority of subjects have been Caucasian males. Given genetic and environmental variability, there are real needs to establish dosing guidelines for ethnic minorities such as the Spanish speaking, as well as to profile any side-effect issues. As Lin points out, there have been rapid population shifts in the United States, as high as 25 percent in the 1990 census, involving people from ethnic minority backgrounds.

The psychotherapist working in managed care must pay attention to drug effects on Spanish-speaking clients in order to work closely with treating psychiatrists regarding adverse side effects of medications. The chemistry of these drugs is complex and affects both antidepressants and neuroleptics (antipsychotic drugs). Lin points out that results with tricyclic antidepressants such as nortriptyline are still inconclusive among Mexican Americans, for example, when compared with Caucasians. Cultural factors in addition to the twenty different enzymes involved in breaking down the psychiatric medications have to be taken into account. As early as 1969, transcultural psychiatrist H. B. Murphy hypothesized that culturally determined normative personality traits would significantly influence the outcome of psychopharmacology treatment. He suggested that if culture gave a strong emphasis to independence, struggle, and action, then patients with cultural backgrounds that emphasize interdependence and social adaptation would require less medication. In fact, personality traits can significantly influence a patient's drug effects. A passive patient under such medication might respond in an expected manner with sedation. In contrast, a person who is athletically inclined and typically action-oriented might show a paradoxical reaction with an increase in agitation, tension, and anxiety.

Lin points out that different cultures, too, influence the type and level of stress and structure and function of social networks. Sadly, as I found out in teaching the anger management class to Spanish-speaking immigrants, few in an average class of ten had much less social support or far fewer relatives or friends to call upon to help them appraise situations that provoked them to anger. Such individuals, if prescribed medications, are less likely to be compliant. In my interactions each week with managed care clients, I routinely inquire into the effects of their psychiatric medications and if they are being taken regularly.

Other researchers find that cultural differences in family atmosphere also contribute to the drug effect. Expressed emotion is a phrase used to characterize the frequent criticism, hostility, and emotional overinvolvement of family members with a psychiatric patient. Latino families tend to have significantly lower expressed emotions compared to Americans and generally are found to need lower doses of antipsychotic medications. This is not always the case, however. As mentioned in Chapter 2, herbal medicines are pharmacologically active and can cause significant interactions with prescribed psychiatric drugs. The psychotherapist needs to inquire about any herbal medicines that the client may be taking.

Despite the fact that psychoactive medication is a major aspect of psychiatric care and crucial in brief psychotherapy treatments, there are repeated reports of cross-national and cross-cultural variations in dosing practices, as well as the side-effect profiles that are associated with these medicines since the 1960s. American psychiatric patients, according to Lin, Poland, and Anderson (1995), seem to require twice as much of these medicines than Europeans for similar clinical effects. Major differences in the process of metabolism are noted among ethnic groups in response to such medications. Nonbiological factors, too, influence the way an individual responds to medications. These include personality, compliance factors, placebo effects, stress, social support, and the prescription style of the physician. Culture also strongly influences the type and level of stress as well as the structure and function of social networks. These are thought to be important factors affecting the prognosis and outcome of treatment of the mentally ill (see World Health Organization 1986).

Since the mid-twentieth century, social scientists have shown how culture and biology interact with each other. When it comes to the effectiveness of psychiatric medication, we see how important it is for the psychotherapist to keep abreast of this research and to be a proactive member of the treatment team, to gently remind the psychiatrist or family physician when necessary to recognize that while one dosage level of a medicine may be viewed as subclinical in some circumstances, it may carry a walloping punch in others.

REBELLIOUS TEENS

It is not unusual for a Latino client to bring a teenage daughter or son to the therapist to "fix" the child. Here we often find issues of acculturation discord, as the children rapidly integrate into the host society and often find their parents' values and rules no longer acceptable. Szapocznik and Kurtines (1993) have examined this problem in some detail with Cuban families in Florida, but their findings are also helpful in Latino clinical practice elsewhere in the United States. Among Latino families, parents and children are exposed to both Latino and mainstream values and customs. Parents tend to remain more attached to traditions, and a classic challenge or family struggle is not unusual in which the children try to obtain autonomy at the same time that their elders try hard to continue family connectedness. Acculturation differences across generations exacerbate these issues, and children lose emotional and social support from the families at the same time that parents lose their position of leadership.

Szapocznik and Kurtines (1993) point out that the parents become unable to manage their children, who are making strong claims for autonomy and who do not accept traditional Latino ways. Thus, it is not unusual to find conduct problems emerging in adolescence. These authors argue for the need to enhance bicultural skills for both parents and their children and to reframe some of the problems in a helpful manner. Among the parents with whom I work, I use the metaphor of the parent bird feeding the young ones in the nest from its own beak. But, as time progresses, the bird literally kicks the other birds out of the nest. I even point to an imaginary nest in the tree outside my office and reiterate the role of the parent in helping the child achieve autonomy to help reframe the rebellion as the natural order of things. It is important to emphasize the communality between parents and their children and deemphasize intergenerational differences. The therapist has to work hard to get the parents to accept and understand the value of certain aspects of American culture embraced by their children. On some occasions, when the child's behavior is beyond the pale, I discuss with the parents the possibility of sending the child to stay with relatives in Mexico in a *rancho* to help motivate the child's future cooperation. I did this in the case of Miguel, an overindulged child who thought the world owed him everything. He came home drunk on several occasions and almost broke an expensive television that his mother's live-in boyfriend had politely asked him not to use. The man left the home in exasperation over the continuing misbehavior of the boy and his mother's inability to control him. Consuela, his mother, eventually sent Miguel to a grandparent in a remote area of Mexico to help him see the light. In this instance, as she informed me some months later, the teen returned much more tractable. In other cases, as with Cuban clients, it may be impossible to send the child back to the "old country," but among Mexican clients this is an alternative worth considering.

Another important issue is that of the gang girl, or *chola*. I have learned to recognize makeup and eyebrow painting as a sign of teen rebelliousness in terms of a youth's personal identity. Harris (1987) has written about 600 gangs that operate in the Los Angeles area. Although Mexican-American gangs have existed for over seventy years and females have been active during that time, today we see more immigrant children joining gangs as a perceived way to obtain more independence from traditional parents. As Harris shows, members identify closely with their neighborhood and often tattoo the name on themselves. These tattoos are so insidious that they even appear on gang members' faces.

One gang member, Dean, had a distinctive tattoo near his eyebrow. This became a handicap for him in trying to get his daughter back from a social services placement with foster parents after the police raided his mother's home where he lived, along with his wife and children and his brother. The brother, also a gang member, lived in the garage and "cooked" speed. The family law judge found it hard to believe that Dean was unaware of what was going on right before his eyes, and the tattoo did not help much either. Harris argues that for core members of gangs, the group is a total institution similar to a military unit, which completely absorbs the individual into the subculture. Members acknowledge that the gang takes precedence over the family. Harris finds that the gang is the most prevalent peer group association in the barrio, the one most readily available and attractive to the children of immigrants, who often rebel against isolation and the rigid rules of their parents.

AIDS

A discussion of clinical issues in the immigrant community would not be complete without a look at AIDS. Traditional *curanderos* in the United States in highly populated Hispanic areas often view AIDS as an illness that they cannot treat, despite the fact that the Centers for Disease Control estimates that as many as 15.5 percent of all AIDS cases in the United States are among Hispanics (cited in Rivera, 1990). *Botanicas,* or shops that sell herbs and folk medicine, are found throughout the United States, wherever immigrants reside. Many of these shops, as Rivera found, sell remedies as well as herbs, candles, perfumes, incense, sprays, etc. One Mexican *curandero* interviewed by Rivera believed that AIDS was related to the folk illness *mal aire,* which can afflict both adults and children. *Mal aire* is believed to be caused by a breeze or wind in a cold climate. At night such air is especially dangerous and is often associated with witchcraft. The illness is thought to enter the body through air manipulated by a witch. In the Latino immigrant families studied by Bulnes (personal communication), parents appear to prefer that their son commit a murder rather than admit that he acquired AIDS through homosexual activities. The *botanica* owners in the United States view AIDS as an incurable illness. AIDS clients are subject to a good deal of AIDS education in Spanish in the media, which precludes its integration into the folk medical beliefs of the Southwest. From the point of view of brief psychotherapy with Latino immigrants, these clients are generally referred to nonprofit health care agencies under special contract.

Numerous researchers have argued that there is a serious lack of information about AIDS and the transmission of HIV among large numbers of Latinos. At a time in the early 1990s when they made up 7.8 percent of the U.S. population, Latinos accounted for 15 percent of the total AIDS cases diagnosed in the country.

Chapter 7

Alcohol, Tuberculosis, and the Spanish-Speaking Immigrant

Mexico, as a nation, has major problems with alcohol abuse, although per capita alcohol consumption throughout Latin America is lower than in the United States (Weissman, 1994). Immigrants from rural and urban regions of that country often bring their dysfunctional patterns of alcohol use and abuse with them to the United States. A recent study found that Mexican Americans, for example, have a lifetime prevalence of 23 percent for alcoholism, similar to other groups from European, American, or Asian societies. While Mexican women often remain in bad marriages when their husbands are alcoholic due to their economic dependence on their spouses, immigrant women appear to be less tolerant of the negative effects of alcoholism on their families' well-being. In recent years, women have become more assertive in dealing with the problems of the alcoholic spouse. They have many more options for employment and are quick to seek EAP assistance or counseling to help them to make decisions and to assuage their guilt about breaking up the family.

Relatively few men appear voluntarily for alcohol treatment. Many are pushed to do so by concerned wives who are not willing to tolerate physical abuse and the expenditure of scarce resources. Of the anger management clients whom I see for ten sessions mandated by the courts, a good 15 percent of the men are arrested for a nondomestic violence incident while under the influence of alcohol. Often they are obliged to attend Alcoholics Anonymous meetings along with anger management classes.

Leticia is a good example of a Latina woman unwilling to permit her husband to continue drinking. She initially sought help for what she thought would be a transition—moving out of her rented room with her two children to avoid nasty encounters with her drunken husband. When José realized that Leticia was serious, he made a vow to give up drinking and the couple was able to rekindle their relationship.

Some patients who have alcoholic and abusive husbands access help through employee assistance programs at work. Marcia came in fearful that her alcoholic husband would kill her and her children, and the therapy hour was spent in arranging access to a shelter. Rarely do these clients return, and the therapist's job is like that of a traffic officer—getting adequate communication going, and an immediate referral to a shelter, as in Marcia's case. Since the Spanish-speaking client often is not aware of community resources outside of his or her particular personal experiences, the psychotherapist's role is psycho-educational in nature, and he or she must explain how such organizations operate and their expectations of the client as well.

Among many of the couples who come into therapy, both husband and wife work. It is not unusual to find the woman's income close to or better than her husband's. Women have more options for employment in urban areas, and often the greater struggle of the men to provide for their families in their marginal positions propels them to seek solace through drinking and the friendship of their barroom companions. Anthropologists can contribute to understanding the cultural spin placed on alcohol use and abuse by using what we call an emic approach. Rather than imposing any model based on white, middle-class norms concerning drinking behavior or even one predicated upon social class membership, an emic approach views the phenomenon of alcohol use from within the context of ethnic group membership.

In the late 1970s, I conducted research on alcohol use among Southern Californian immigrants. This chapter examines some of the major ways in which alcohol poses a problem for the Spanish-speaking immigrant, and the kinds of techniques that can be used successfully to treat the disease. The ethnographic method, which employs participant observation, general community interaction, interviewing, obtaining informants' life histories, and diaries, has always yielded important data in many areas of group behavior. The anthropologist has always been concerned with the way in which people set up rules and categories and code and define their experience. From a holistic perspective, it is important to understand the way in which alcohol acts as a means of accommodation to problems created by conflicting cultural or racial patterns as they precipitate alcohol use.

With the late Dr. Daniel Feldman and funded by the National Institute of Alcoholism and Alcohol Abuse, I conducted a cartographic examination of the drinking milieu in the county where I work (de Rios and Feldman, 1976, 1977). Experienced informants helped me map the drinking milieu, and I examined the iconic, emblematic, and expressive elements associated with alcohol. I interviewed bartenders, waitresses, liquor sales personnel, and others who were in frequent contact with the Spanish-speaking drinking population. Many recurrent patterns emerged.

Before I talk about ways in which the therapist can help the Spanish-speaking client who suffers from alcohol abuse, it is important to understand some of the sociological implications of alcohol use patterns. Often, immigrants do not consider drinking a problem when an Anglo would. Alcoholics, too, are viewed quite differently by members of the immigrant community compared to Anglos. Immigrant payoffs in drinking may be fundamentally different from those held to be operational in the larger society. Stress related to discrimination, prejudice, and the trauma of migration are important factors that justify alcohol use and abuse as a suitable cultural response to a person's inner tensions. Thus, after a hard week's work, drinking alcohol on weekends is not uncommon as a coping mechanism among many of my clients' husbands.

Olinda, a young Ecuadorian woman, came to see me for marriage counseling. Her husband, Fernando, drank twelve cans of beer or more each Friday and Saturday night, either at home or out with friends. They fought constantly, and Fernando did not recognize that he had a drinking problem. Like many Latin Americans, he did not see beer as a *vicio* (vice), and he did not know what all the fuss was about. On further prodding, Fernando realized that if he did not diminish his drinking, he would lose his wife and children.

Many immigrant drinkers, such as Camacho, take their alcohol quietly at home and avoid bars. Even Camacho knew that things were not going well for him. His children were doing poorly in school, his wife was distraught, and he was beginning to have problems with his liver. In therapy, he told about his on-again, off-again love affair with a married co-worker who was badly abused by her husband. By working on cognitive techniques of rational problem solving, the stress on Camacho lessened and he stopped drinking. He felt a very strong loyalty to his wife and children, however, and realized by himself that he had to make a decision about continuing with this other woman at work or remaining with his family.

It is important to understand how a segment of the immigrant community may self-medicate depression and anxiety with alcohol and present in psychotherapy with a dual diagnosis. To further complicate the analysis, many barrios that have large numbers of Spanish-speaking immigrants also may be listed among individual county poverty areas. Some or all of the drinking behavior that characterizes the immigrant is also a function of being poor.

In the course of my research, I visited bars, chosen by resource consultants, that were representative of the bars available in several Spanish-speaking communities. These visits were often made on weekend evenings and allowed me to make a preliminary map of the drinking environment. Analysis showed that Spanish-surname alcohol abusers did not appear in any significant numbers within county alcohol rehabilitation referrals by the courts. Rather, many were arrested for alcohol-related crimes. At the time of my study, a large percentage of inmates in the county jail (28 to 34 percent) were Spanish-speaking, which may indicate that Latino alcohol abusers are incarcerated rather than rehabilitated. I contacted a long-term county hospital facility in the region and was able to spend two and a half months interviewing Mexican nationals who were inpatients in their tuberculosis ward. Approximately two-thirds of these patients were heavy users of alcohol.

I found that the bar/drinking milieu served as a voluntary association and social brokerage for the acculturating, translocated rural peasantry. Sociological studies of voluntary associations showed that Spanish-speaking groups are much less likely than Anglos or blacks to participate in these clublike groupings (Williams, 1973). In situations of acculturation, the drinking milieu functions as a setting in which cultural learning occurs. The enormous variation between bar settings that I observed correlates with the commonality of clientele and interests in specific drinking settings. The immigrant faces many new dilemmas as a peasant translocated to the city. The drinking milieu becomes an educational network and social learning center where the immigrant can become acquainted with the demands, rules, and expectations of the larger society. Voluntary associations function to adapt the immigrant to the new urban environment. With increased modernization, industrialization, urbanization, and the concomitant large-scale rural-urban migrations, kinship and territory are no longer effective means to reorganize the immigrant's existing networks. Common-interest associations serve a number of functions and act as adaptive mechanisms in situations of change. Given the paucity of formal club-organizational groupings among Latinos, the Spanish-speaking bar is like a library or employment office.

In my research, I found it interesting that in the county studied, there was no skid row phenomenon. One interview I had with a fifty-two-year-old Spanish "wino" showed that he had ongoing family support over the last ten years, even though he was a derelict and socially irresponsible. The difficulty in finding a discernible Spanish-speaking alcohol-derelict population is most likely related to the way that the family springs into play to protect its members, particularly those who are problem drinkers. The mechanism of denial with regard to alcohol abuse continues to be prominent within the Spanish-speaking immigrant family when confronted with the presence of addictive drinking by a family member. The family acts in a protective way, whenever possible, to buffer the alcoholic against punishments meted out by the larger society.

A study of alcoholism prevalence in a southern Texas clinic and the utilization of medical services by Latinos found that the prevalence rate of alcoholism was similar to that among men from other ethnic backgrounds. More men than women suffered from this disorder. Interestingly, if these findings can be generalized, alcoholic patients were more often unemployed or disabled, which impacts the managed care patient base and accounts for the smaller number of patients who present with this problem (Caetano, 1989).

One consistently elicited theme that I see again and again among Spanish-speaking managed care patients with alcohol problems deals with an adult male's personal decision to seek a pattern of sobriety as a response to his perceived excessive drinking. A *juramento* (vow) given before God or the Virgin is cited to dismiss any family concerns that the client will return to drinking. Generally, perceptions of abusive drinking come from the drinkers themselves rather than spouses, children, employers, family members, or friends. In local shelters for battered women, 94 percent of the Latina women had battering partners who used alcohol. Half of the men also used illegal drugs such as cocaine and marijuana (Sullivan, 1992). The concept and value of the macho as a mature and responsible adult is said to be negated through lack of free will, or *voluntad*. The individual chooses to be irresponsible in his continued abusive drinking.

For rehabilitation, medical detoxification programs are generally preferred over those stressing social detoxification. Most mental health hospitals contracted by managed care companies that I have seen simply are not set up to provide treatment in Spanish for the monolingual client. A week or ten days' stay is often the maximum time that such clients spend inside a facility. However, case managers often can be prevailed upon to permit multiple outpatient therapy sessions during subsequent weeks to help the client get the most therapeutic benefit from the detoxification process.

Rouse, Carter, and Rodriguez-Andrew (1995) found that sociocultural factors do impact alcoholism rates. Sociocultural groups such as Latino immigrants can differ in rates of inner tension and anxiety and the need for relief of such tension and anxiety as well as in attitudes toward drinking. Women alcoholics, for example, experience more anxiety, more depression, and more opposition to treatment than do men. These authors see alcohol addiction in Latino and other minority women as inextricably intertwined with issues of racism, sexism, unemployment, poverty, and substandard housing and child care services.

In a 1984 survey funded by the National Institute on Alcohol Abuse and Alcoholism (Caetano, 1989), alcohol use among Latinos was examined, and researchers found a high abstinence rate among women (47 percent) and a high rate of heavy drinking among men (36 percent). While in the general population men tended to decrease their alcohol consumption between the ages of twenty and forty, Cervantes and colleagues (1990) found Latino men continued to experience high levels of alcohol use and alcohol-related problems well into their forties. Latinos born in the United States, moreover, were more likely to be heavy drinkers than foreign-born Latino drinkers. Caetano's (1989) study of alcohol and drug use within racial and ethnic groups shows that Latin American women, largely from South and Central America, had the highest rates of abstention. Immigrant men reported a different pattern of alcohol consumption, low frequency but high quantity. After they immigrated, their drinking changed to both high frequency and high quantity.

It is useful to inquire about drinking patterns in the household of the family that you are counseling, even if this is not mentioned as a presenting problem in the initial clinical interview. Moreover, Latinos are more likely to access treatment as involuntary rather than as voluntary clients. Rouse, Carter, and Rodriguez-Andrew (1995) point out that direct questioning, however, may not be useful in establishing the existence of an alcohol problem or addiction. Rather, they suggest a friendly conversation, which can be more effective in determining the desired mental health status or clinical condition.

USEFUL INTERVENTION TECHNIQUES FOR THE LATINO ALCOHOLIC CLIENT

As with all clients who have chemical dependency problems, motivation is an important factor in treatment. An occasional EAP or short-term referral may come in as the result of a supervisor's initiative. In one case, Pablo was very anxious to get rid of his methamphetamine and alcohol addiction because he was engaged to the boss's daughter. He believed that he had a good future in the factory where he worked if he could only maintain his sobriety.

Polcin (1995), in an important article on alcohol intervention that has implications for the Latino patient, discusses the many consequences of alcohol abuse. They include family dysfunction, high arrest and incarceration rates, health problems, and economic costs related to employee absenteeism and poor work performance. Latino immigrants have special needs. The use of alcohol as a coping mechanism has existed in these communities in Latin America for hundreds of years (see Helzer and Canino, 1992). We know that the Aztec and Maya cultures used intoxicants and hallucinogens as part of religious rituals for millennia (de Rios, 1984a). Fabrega (1995) points out that the Western health model of alcoholism as a disorder shows little understanding of cultural variations in how alcohol is used and how excessive drinking is conceptualized and handled.

To treat the Latino immigrant patient who presents with issues of alcohol dependency, Polcin (1997) argues for the use of cognitive behavioral techniques combined with a twelve-step Alcoholics Anonymous program, which can be very effective. We need to change dysfunctional behaviors and to help the client identify the social situations that trigger, fuel, rationalize, and reinforce substance use. Emotional issues and interpersonal conflicts can be identified to help the client learn new techniques, new ways of thinking, and new behavioral skills. Rational-emotive therapy is helpful in teaching the client to give up the need to be perfect and to stop finding disasters everywhere. Most Latinos do best with a commitment to abstinence.

The typical journal homework assignments used in cognitive therapies are not useful as many immigrant clients are not particularly fond of writing. Many have a sixth-grade education or less. Rather, the client needs to assess the trigger that precipitates drinking episodes. For example, José's work in construction inevitably led to his being paid in a bar, since he had to wait for his boss to give him a ride home. He found himself drinking all the time, even when he really did not want to. The client had to learn to identify his feelings and thoughts in response to provocations to drink.

Among many of the anger management clients I see, abstinence is commonplace, especially after people have experienced the effects of aversive conditioning by spending time in jail or separating from their spouses due to their angry explosions while drunk. Manuel now regrets those many times when he turned to alcohol. His wife left him alone with three children after he beat her. He was obliged to spend two months in jail. Therapists must teach their clients to practice new behaviors, to inhibit drinking, to learn new strategies to use when they feel like drinking, and how to recognize and avoid situations, people, and places that are triggers to drinking. They also need to learn about options to practice when they are not able to avoid these cues.

Polcin (1997) suggests that we teach the client to use a scale from 1 to 100 to measure the craving to drink. As with many behavior modification techniques, before we can change behavior we must bring it out of the unconscious realm to the light of day. Scaling a craving for alcohol is used as a substitute for an immediate drink. By scaling the craving for alcohol, individuals learn to provide themselves with positive self-talk and ask themselves, "How badly do I want a drink in this situation?" It is imperative to teach clients to tolerate their alcohol cravings without acting on them. The Spanish-language relaxation tape discussed in Chapter 3 can be helpful to restore some degree of control to the individual who is tense and upset. Using AA techniques such as calling upon a sober friend to support one's own sobriety, as well as avoiding situations that trigger cravings, is simple good sense. When people are in situations where they feel overwhelmed by a desire to drink, it is good to state that they themselves have decided to leave. No one makes them leave, and they decide what is the adult and healthy thing to do.

There is a real need to challenge patients' cognitions that fuel drinking. If people think they need to drink to relax, to socialize, to cope with stress, or that all their friends drink and that is the only way to have fun—these self-statements are inaccurate distortions and trigger alcohol use. The therapist must challenge them, and clients must learn how to consider how their cognitions are distorted and to restate them more accurately. Clients respond very well to stress reduction skills as a substitution for drinking. Assertiveness training (see Appendix B) or teaching communication and good listening skills also can be helpful.

I use a problem-solving technique, brainstorming, which examines all possible responses to a given problem that the client faces. After spelling out all the alternatives (on a blackboard, or by pencil and paper), the potential benefits and consequences of each choice can be listed. This controls impulsivity and teaches clients to develop possible options and to consider consequences before they decide on any action.

One can also teach clients to refuse to drink by stating or disclosing to others that they are recovering alcoholics. I tell my clients the story about how I left a really good party once, with conga dancing that I was enjoying, because the host was an alcoholic and wanted everyone else to get drunk along with him. Role-playing can be useful in rehearsing some of these tactics, especially if they are new to the client. Of course, we have to instruct clients to throw away all the liquor in the house and to develop a list of sober friends whom they can call upon in an emergency, as well as to join a twelve-step support group to deal with their feelings of guilt and shame to prevent further drinking.

Many studies talk about the importance of triggers—the bar, old friends, etc.—and the need to develop a new and different lifestyle to avoid temptation. All of the client's underlying problems must be dealt with, such as negative moods, depression, or other dual diagnostic issues. The client must be helped in vocational planning and to resolve relationship issues. Latinos respond very well to the disease model of alcoholism. This approach is useful with people who are not psychologically sophisticated. Clients quickly learn to appreciate their absolution from blame and guilt. Participation in AA meetings helps people become aware of their lack of power over alcohol, which propels their lives into disarray. The RET program can help to challenge distorted thoughts that fuel alcohol use, particularly the irrational belief that the world must be a perfect place and meet one's immediate needs now.

THE TUBERCULOSIS PATIENT

Links between alcoholism and tuberculosis are hardly new, as heavy drinkers generally lose their appetite and often take poor physical care of themselves. As part of my early research in Latino alcohol use, I also conducted interviews on a tuberculosis ward among nineteen Spanish-speaking men who were Mexican immigrants to Southern California (de Rios and Feldman, 1976, 1977). They ranged in age from twenty to fifty-three years. The majority of them were undocumented, mostly monolingual workers. The reason they gave for immigrating was to search for work. Their average schooling was five years per person, and a few were illiterate. Fifty percent had experienced poverty during childhood. The majority were not married. When asked about the effects of alcohol, they reported that drinking made them peaceful and quiet, brave, obstreperous, bad tempered, high, violent, irritable, argumentative, and unable to accept authority. They said that alcohol caused them to live in a fantasy, to have a big mouth, to be jealous, to fight with their wives, and to provide them relief from social pressure and tensions.

Patients were aware of both negative and positive aspects of drinking. They were sophisticated in understanding the association of their alcohol use with their nutritional problems, such as diminished appetite and weight loss, as well as other difficulties that led them to contract tuberculosis. Almost half of the sample had fathers who drank heavily during their childhood. Prior to contracting tuberculosis, ten men used alcohol on a daily basis, three occasionally, one seldom, and five not at all. Most drank beer and preferred drinking mainly in bars, but also with friends, at parties, at relatives' homes, or at work. Men began to drink at about fifteen years of age. The research showed a link between moderate to heavy drinking and tuberculosis for stressed, migrating men. People found that drinking gave them relief from stressors as well as permission to engage in certain types of behavior. The Spanish-speaking immigrants whom I studied found in alcohol consumption relief from stress, which inured them to problems resulting from acculturation. Many patients had lived in poverty and were poorly prepared for life in the United States, from an educational and occupational perspective.

Recent epidemiological studies show that since the time of my early research on tuberculosis, the declining incidence of tuberculosis in the United States has reversed, and there has been a resurgence of cases. From 1986 to 1993, for example, the number of diagnosed cases of active tuberculosis among foreign-born patients increased from 22 to 30 percent. Most of the foreign-born patients with tuberculosis were from Latin America. Rates for Latinos are four times higher than those of native residents. I have seen several children referred for psychotherapy who have tested positively for tuberculosis, and there continues to be a high relative rate of tuberculosis among foreign-born children (McKenna, McCray, and Onorato, 1995). Since the tiredness, listlessness, and fatigue experienced by patients who suffer from tuberculosis can mirror symptoms of depression, it is important to rule out such problems and suggest tuberculosis screening of the client's family if a physician has not already done so. Although tuberculosis has diminished as a health hazard in the United States, the psychotherapist working with the Latino immigrant client must be ready to rule this disease out of any evaluation of the client.

Chapter 8

Maria, the Murderer, and the Misogynist

In this chapter, I present a detailed case study of a family I treated over seven sessions, to illustrate some of the concepts described in this book. While I expected that my language skills and interest in Latino culture from my fieldwork experiences with traditional folk healers in Peru would be useful to me as a therapist, it was not until I met Maria at a child guidance clinic and worked with her and her family that I realized just how very committed I would become to working with Latino clients. I extended my interests from drug-induced altered states of consciousness in the Peruvian Amazon to hypnosis and metaphor.

THE CASE

Maria came into the clinic very tearful and upset. Her second oldest child, a boy of thirteen, ran away from home after she had slapped him hard to discipline him and bruised his face. He was found by the police and placed in temporary foster care. Social services mandated family therapy in order for family reconciliation to occur. Maria's depression was quite severe, far greater than the events warranted. In fact, the boy was very quickly reunited with her, returning home after a few weeks. As she told me her history, I became very connected to her story, as it reminded me of the many sad and woeful tales I had documented in my year in the Amazon living among the urban poor (de Rios 1972, 1984a). As Polster and Polster (1973, p. 187) suggest in their studies of Gestalt psychotherapy, "every person's life is worth a novel," and Maria's was right up there with regard to pathos and misery.

In southern Mexico, Maria, at the age of fourteen, caught the eye of an aggressive, violent laborer who had murdered a man. He kidnapped her and fled northward. She lived with him for several years and bore him three children. Her life was full of misery, as the man was an alcoholic and was both physically and verbally abusive to her. At times she worked as an itinerant peddler in order to feed her children. Eventually she was able to leave him and migrate to the United States. She lived with an older man for several years who protected her, and she bore him one child. Later, Maria separated from him and was on her own for a while, until she met Jorge, her current common-law husband. At the time that she entered psychotherapy, they had a little boy who was four years old. Jorge and Maria argued a good deal, although the couple seemed to have a strong, loving bond and relationship.

I saw Maria intermittently in therapy for seven visits, always subject to the health of her car. A number of developments affected her. At first, obtaining a history was very traumatic for her, as she had suffered enormous hardships in her life, now capped by "losing her son." Moreover, away from her extended kinship unit in Mexico and with no desire to return, she had few friends or confidants and was not at all psychologically sophisticated. She had never told her history to a stranger or even a friend.

At first, to satisfy the mandate of the abuse situation, I taught Maria behavioral modification techniques to replace the harsh disciplining style that she took for granted in rearing her children, prior to her son's running away. I had observed this type of harsh parent-child interaction among many urban poor people. Nonetheless, parents such as Maria, with strong bonds of love and concern for their children, often are willing to learn new ways to respond. Her son was converted to a Jehovah's Witness by the foster family where he was placed, and some issues involved were to bring this to the attention of Social Services and actually to hasten the reunification process.

Although Maria was referred for medication and began a trial of antidepressant medications, she clearly needed to learn some relaxation techniques. I utilized the hypnotic induction discussed in Chapter 3. Several cultural elements were involved that set the induction apart from what I had learned in my psychology class in hypnosis in 1978. I fondly remembered how tactile I found Latino culture to be. I often joked with my students that during the entire year that I lived in the Amazon, I was obliged to give an *abrazo* and kiss the post office lady who sold me stamps! In the induction, by asking clients to move "energy" slowly into their bodies, incrementally, from the top of the head to the shoulders (covering all bases, e.g., cheek, jaw relaxing, mouth opening, neck muscles relaxing, etc.), and then on through the body, to the feet, I found that a focused state of awareness generally ensued, especially among trauma patients, who responded very well to parasympathetic toning after the hypervigilance that typically followed the trauma (de Rios and Friedman, 1990). I made a gift of the relaxation tape to Maria and personalized it to meet her specific needs. I prepared a script that included geographical imagery familiar to her from Mexico. This helped to establish a strong therapeutic alliance with her.

Maria complained bitterly about her current spouse *(marido)*—this term is used to indicate a common-law relationship. Jorge was very clearly biased with regard to his own son, and neglectful and disinterested in Maria's four other children. Jorge took his son on special outings and indulged him with candy and toys. Although he was not mean or abusive to the other children, he basically ignored them. I met with Jorge alone on two occasions. Frankly, I did not expect to learn much or even to be particularly successful in getting him to open up to me. Much to my surprise, after some initial queries as to where he grew up, how he met Maria, his migratory experiences coming to the United States, etc., a very important cultural theme emerged that helped me to understand the major source of conflict between him and Maria.

Jorge grew up in a *ranchito,* a hamlet of perhaps twenty to thirty families. As with other Mexican men of similar rural background, he made a distinction between a *señorita* (read virgin) and a *mujer* (woman). This value was instilled in Jorge at a very early age. I remember an incident in Peru, when I was in my late twenties and accompanying the local Amazon soccer team to a rural hamlet for a match. A drunken man accosted me while I was with my hosts and became very aggressive. The couple with whom I was traveling said to the drunk, "She is a señorita," and he moved away quickly, shamed by his blunder.

For the rural Mexican farmer to marry well, he must obtain his own señorita. Indeed, Jorge migrated to the United States simply to earn enough money to pay for a forthcoming wedding, a house, and furnishings. Unfortunately, the woman married another man. Jorge was desolate. Then he met Maria, who had had not only one *marido,* but two, and a pack of children to boot. His dream of a virgin bride was destroyed, but he agreed to take on the responsibility of supporting the woman and her children. After a time, at least, he had his son, and he was not an unkind stepfather.

One of the therapeutic tasks I had to deal with was to help Jorge recognize that Maria's children were part of the "package deal" that accompanied her, and that it was unfair of him to ask her to distance herself emotionally from her children. At that time, the theme of the "evil stepparent" in Mexican culture became very clear to me and gave me insight into a cultural value and belief that has been very helpful in conducting subsequent family therapy with Latino families over the years.

Because of the value placed on virginity and chastity in rural Mexican culture, and the fragility of the relationship bond between common-law spouses, mature women have particular cultural stressors when they unite with a new boyfriend, who is often unable emotionally to deal with the woman's children, who are daily reminders of her lack of "virtue" in this particular cultural milieu. Subsequent cases I have treated often involved men and women who as children were sent off to their maternal grandparents to be raised because of their mother's discomfort at having the children of a former *marido* present, almost as if it were salt in a wound. This cultural theme had to be addressed with Jorge and Maria, since no grandparents were available to pick up the slack, and the success of the couple's relationship indeed hinged on Jorge's commitment to the family unit. His misogynist stance was very provocative and created repercussions with his eldest stepdaughter.

Maria's oldest daughter, Elena, at the time of our meeting was fifteen years old. She functioned effectively as a "child nurse." As with many poverty-stricken families in Latin America, the oldest child often had major responsibilities for child care for other siblings, particularly the youngest one. Elena was in high school and wanted to be with her friends, to shop, to eat pizza, etc., and to act like any other American teenager. Her mother, Maria, had other ideas and, perhaps in reaction to her own experiences and traumatic memories, closeted the girl at home and was very indignant and unhappy at Elena's complaints and rudeness. Needless to say, by Maria's standards she was doing a good job, since the girl was almost past the age when she would have been encouraged to marry as a virgin had she remained in the Mexican hamlet. Given the importance of chastity as a cultural theme, it is a good idea to marry off a daughter at age fourteen or fifteen, before the imperious sex drives result in loss of virtue. Elena, on the other hand, was a typical Southern California teenager and felt caged and oppressed by her child care duties, her mother's attempts to control her, and a lack of discretionary spending money in the household.

To help Maria gain some control over the family situation, we had a meeting with all five children in the clinic conference room. The children were very excited about the meeting and we used a "good kid chart" (see Daily Duties, Appendix B), available in pads. One chart would be set up for each child, listing the tasks and rewards for the child. In turn, each child participated to the best of his or her ability to design the tasks around the house that needed to be performed and his or her particular role in the household. With Spanish-speaking families, especially those who live at the poverty level, it is easy to use metaphors of collaboration and cooperation because children have often known hunger and want and recognize the need for such cooperation. The children responded very well to the reward schedules to recognize good behavior that we set up, within the limits of Maria's meager budget. Since rural farming people such as Maria were reared with an authoritarian pattern, it is not generally easy for them to respond to a STEP-type program that focuses on the logical consequences of behavior and democratic themes (Dinkemayer, McKay, and Dinkmeyer, 1997). The children, however, recognized a real ally in the therapist, who might help them gain some autonomy and input into household rules and resource distribution.

Around this time, Jorge's seventeen-year-old brother, Pedro, came to live with the family to earn money to send to his parents in Mexico. He lost his job and began to spend a good deal of time around the house. Maria was very upset because she caught Pedro hiding in a closet and spying on Elena emerging seminude from the bathroom after a shower. Maria was fearful that the child's stepuncle would rape her, which provoked memories of her own traumatic teenage years. Jorge was very noncommittal about this threat and was unwilling to speak to his brother or make any changes at home. As part of my role as an educator as well as therapist, I pointed out the difference in state-level controls on family life in the United States compared to Mexico. When Jorge realized that all the children might be taken from the home if sexual abuse were suspected (that is, he might lose his own son as well), he responded very quickly, "reading the riot act" to his brother and threatening to send him back to Mexico if he did not behave more prudently and with respect. Jorge's misogynist attitude had clearly influenced his younger brother.

Resolution of this case was not neat and clean. The clinic lost its contract with the county. Several of the therapists, including me, were laid off, and clients such as Maria were transferred to another clinic that had received the new contract for short-term service. Toward the end of the sessions at the original clinic, Maria had another setback when Elena ran away to live with her seventeen-year-old boyfriend. The relationship between Jorge and Maria softened, and Jorge began to be more compassionate with the children. He never became a strong father figure for them, but he began to consider them in his activities and planning. Maria's depression lifted and she was able to obtain a factory job, adding to their family income, enabling her to buy a dependable used car and to fight less with her children over money. She called me a year later and wanted to resume psychotherapy to talk again, but circumstances did not permit it.

THE THERAPY PROCESS:
THE CLIENT

One of the most dramatic issues for me with regard to this case had to do with the therapy process itself. Rural farmers, disenfranchised, living in a society that has experienced more than 400 years of oppression as the result of the Spanish conquest, have neither the time nor the inclination for reflection or introspection. Forced into the clinic by the state in order to regain access to her son, Maria was hardly a person to fit the mold of the "good patient"—young, educated, psychologically savvy, etc. Just the opposite. Balancing this, however, are several factors. No interpreter was necessary for her to experience the psychotherapeutic relationship. The recounting of her history and her own ability to see the pattern and desperation of her life would certainly have shaken a stronger person than she. Yet despite her hardships, she had loving children, a loving husband, and some hope for the future. In response to her needs, the antidepressant medication was timely and effective, lifting Maria's spirits and giving her energy to deal with her problems.

As the sympathetic therapist, I fit the cultural role of an asymmetrical other (e.g., a hacienda owner's wife, a godparent of higher social status), very common in rural Mexico, the model of a person who might intercede on one's behalf in times of strife. The hypnosis tape, which I offered as a gift, as a sign of caring and concern, resonated with meaning for the client, as the empowerment symbols were ego syntonic to the client's needs. Moreover, from an anthropological perspective, gift-giving was elevated to a high art, since anthropologists prefer not to pay for data, but to establish a social relationship with the individuals with whom they interact in order to set up a pattern of reciprocity.

The physical effects of the relaxation therapy were immediate and inspired confidence. The family meetings with the children maintained generational boundaries and reinforced the client's status as parent, while presenting a constructive model for change that was doable and that engaged the enthusiasm of the children. The client's husband began to change his behavior toward her children, creating a more relaxed and loving atmosphere at home. The client's ability eventually to find and keep a job and to buy into the "American dream" was the capstone to it all.

THE THERAPY PROCESS:
THE THERAPIST

What about me? How did this case affect my personal growth? I certainly had compassion and even awe for this woman's ability to survive her own personal history. I remembered vividly the biographies that I had collected among the urban poor when I lived in the Peruvian Amazon—their hardships and trials, their anxieties and concerns. I admired Maria's self-sacrifice and devotion to her children, and I commiserated on the difficulties she encountered in influencing her children. I envied her the intensity of her love for her children and realized how the adversity that she had experienced colored her emotions and passions for her children. I felt tremendous pleasure at being able to help her. She was not from my own ethnic background. I often felt I was in uncharted waters. True, I had married a mestizo man from Peru; true, I had a dark-skinned teenage child, now in high school (much better behaved, thank God, than Maria's); true, I had a stepchild, as Jorge had, and I had to deal with trying to love that child as much I could, even though it was not mine. I even went to the opposite extreme from Jorge and insisted that everything be equal between my daughter and stepdaughter, even when I felt like favoring my own child. Unlike Jorge, I had spent nine years with my husband trying to obtain custody of my stepdaughter, and I even spent a year abroad in Peru, directing an overseas program, which permitted me to petition U.S. Immigration to obtain a visa for my stepdaughter. My anger at Jorge for his disinterest in his stepchildren contrasted with my sense of devotion to my stepdaughter. I had to analyze my own countertransference issues so as not to appear to take sides or be unsympathetic to Jorge's cultural issues regarding his wife's children.

Was some of my countertransference due to my own perception of the prejudice and discrimination problems that my daughters and husband had to face which I, as a white woman, did not? When I married, a WASP colleague of mine said that I should not change my name, that it would be better not to have a Spanish surname in California and bear the brunt of prejudice. Yet, oddly enough, from the perspective of being a psychotherapist, it was a great help to have a Spanish surname when I conducted psychotherapy within the Spanish-speaking community. Did my countertransference mean that I might have been more helpful if I could separate my own quixotic sense of justice from the client's needs? Was I seeing issues that were not really there?

I do know, however, that this case made it very clear to me that I could put my anthropological knowledge to practical use. It is one thing to know about structural aspects of culture and be able to recite a cookbook trait list. But as a psychotherapist, listening to the client, I could induce abstractions from the data I was obtaining as part of my anthropological theoretical framework. I could listen with a "third ear" and emit the empathy and care that directed me to become a therapist in the first place. Hopefully, the same principles that made me a good ethnographer could now help me as a therapist. More important, this dual career track could help me be creative in trying to design and implement interventions that would help Latino clients. As an anthropologist, it was very clear to me that understanding culture consisted of far more than the simple translation of ideas from one culture to another. One really has to understand the configuration or context of beliefs. Understanding the beliefs and values of other people, even when they do not resonate with one's own cultural values and expectations, is a real challenge. What might appear to my feminist instincts to be a negative phenomenon (the virgin bride motif, for example), nonetheless could be utilized to negotiate resolutions of conflicts for clients and to design metaphors and images in hypnotic trance to meet their needs.

In reflecting on this case of Maria, the murderer, and the misogynist, I have wondered how generalizable my personal experience has been. I believe other therapists need to take into account cultural variables in their psychological interventions, and I find myself spending more and more time seeking opportunities to teach nurses, psychotherapists, physicians, and other health personnel in my recognition of the need for synthesis.

In the last chapter, I turn to issues confronting non-Latino psychotherapists who find themselves treating Spanish-speaking immigrant clients.

Chapter 9

The Non-Latino Psychotherapist and the Spanish-Speaking Patient

With the browning of America currently taking place in the United States, whereby one out of four Americans defines himself or herself as an ethnic minority person (U.S. Bureau of the Census, 1991), it is clear that the Latino patient entering psychotherapy probably will be unlikely to encounter a Latino psychotherapist. The field of psychotherapy is in the throes of transformation, as culturally specific therapeutic paradigms and techniques develop to meet the unique sociocultural reality and worldview of distinctive minority groups that all therapists must address (Comas-Diaz, 1992). The lesson from anthropology is that the outsider may have an even greater likelihood of understanding and recording cultural events and meanings of a client than a person so steeped in a culture that boundaries and distinctions fail to emerge. As long as non-Latino psychotherapists are willing to keep an open mind, to be respectful of the roles of family members and community structures, hierarchies, values, and beliefs within the client's culture, they are likely to be effective in treating Latino clients, and can obtain competency in multicultural issues.

The issue of trust is important here. Falicov (1998) discusses the issues of trust as a challenge for therapists who are members of the dominant culture. It is not easy for an outsider to imagine what it is like to live the experiences of the other. The Spanish word *confianza* is a concept of trust that grows as the result of the gradual development of a relationship based on *personalismo*. The therapist, according to Falicov (1998), must be respectful of the client's dignity by communicating kindness, fairness, and basic courtesy and personal interest rather than simply by outcomes. She suggests that the therapist should be open and honest about the clinical setting and the goals of therapy and offer to answer any questions that other family members may have. A confrontational approach is not valued, and small disclosures (such as that you, too, have been a parent), are important to establish a therapeutic alliance. Once *confianza* is established, meeting therapeutic goals truly happens faster.

Some writers, such as Comas-Diaz and Greene (1994), argue that some people of color with a non-middle-class orientation may prefer psychotherapeutic approaches that are directive, offer advice, and work with systems and significant others toward increasing interdependence. Vasquez (1994) points out that therapists face risks of miscommunication in psychotherapy, especially when the client is an ethnic minority female and the therapist is an Anglo-American male. Therapists must recognize how they are influenced by their own socialization—assumptions, values, attitudes, biases, and stereotypes. Such individuals must be constantly vigilant to be free of personal and professional biases. Western values such as rugged individualism, autonomy, competition, progress and future orientation, nuclear family structure, assertiveness, etc., as Vasquez argues, are not universal values. The Latina female may hold different values that emphasize family and group success over individual achievement and may be socialized to maneuver, not assert. In fact, there is no adequate translation for the term "assertiveness training." Therapists, however well-meaning, must not implicitly impose their own values as a measuring stick for Latino clients. Vasquez reiterates how important it is for the clinician to realize that the core components of an individual's identity are gender, ethnicity, and socioeconomic class. A large percentage of Latino immigrants are of lower socioeconomic status, regardless of generational status in the United States.

As we saw in Chapter 2, the therapist must assess and evaluate the Latino patient. He or she must consider the impact of adverse social, environmental, and sociopolitical factors when designing present interventions, as well as accepting what Comas-Diaz (1992) calls "pluralistic paradigms." Torrey (1972), too, argues that shamans do psychotherapy and help people who have problems in living or mental diseases. Different people divide up their worlds differently, as we saw in Chapter 4. However, a certain degree of shared worldview is necessary for successful psychotherapy to occur. It is not just a language barrier that makes cross-cultural psychotherapy difficult, but the cognitive differences between people.

Torrey (1972) finds many ways in which people get well. The expectation of the patient is important, and people who expect to get well are more likely to do so. Shamans and psychologists, according to Torrey, all raise or lower their patients' expectations by the exterior and furnishings of their office, their accessories, paraphernalia, rattles, special masks, couches, or their training and reputations. While therapists and clients who come from the same culture may implicitly share the same cognitive orientation, what is more important is how successful the therapist has been in seeing patients from other subcultures and to what degree he or she values the cultural characteristics of the client. Moreover, to take advantage of the biology of hope, how does that therapist raise the patient's expectations? What is the client's perception of the building where the therapist sees patients? How far does a client come to see the therapist? What paraphernalia does he or she use during the course of treatment? What is the therapist's reputation? Does the therapist take a history? Does he or she prescribe drugs? What conditioning techniques, such as relaxation exercises, does the therapist call upon? Is the family involved in therapy? Does the therapist try to remove symptoms? Does he or she change patients' attitudes and alter behavior? Does the therapist improve a patient's interpersonal relationships? All of these elements and more have to be considered to predict the efficacy of the therapeutic endeavor.

Although some writers liken psychotherapists to witchdoctors or shamans (Torrey, 1972), others such as Gonzalez, Bieves, and Gardner (1973) examine the multicultural perspective in counseling, which provides the opportunity for two people from different cultural perspectives to disagree without one being considered right and the other one wrong. This results in a tolerance and encouragement of diverse and complex perspectives and points to the fact that there is more than one way to arrive at a solution. These authors recognize that the failure to understand or accept another worldview can have detrimental consequences for clients. Brody (1987) sees racial homogeneity for the client and therapist as less important than the bonding thread of interpersonal trust in a same-gender dyad, where a climate of equality is cultivated.

As far as therapeutic intervention goes, the therapist must empower the client to engage in change if he or she decides to do that, emphasizing strengths, not weaknesses. A caring attitude is all-important. The therapist must not encourage a client to adapt to an unhealthy environment but to change it or leave it. At times, the therapist may need to engage in direct advocacy activities and use his or her expertise and knowledge of how various forces affect the mental health of Latinos to educate others.

Psychotherapists are cautioned to view behavior as meaningful when it is linked to cultural learning, expectations, and values. Anthropologists, too, pride themselves on their cultural relativity, just as the social constructionist movement in psychology argues that the meanings of the world are derived from social interactions and emphasizes how people create knowledge and understanding. Multiple outlooks are equally valid. This postmodern paradigm tells us that we must not perpetuate the status quo when working with minority and marginalized clientele. My personal perspective is to see myself as helping the client to become as powerful as possible, first by understanding how systems work and then by deciding what to do to manage and manipulate them appropriately to fully meet the client's needs. The danger in conducting cross-cultural therapy is that there may be discrepancies in the participants' shared assumptions, experiences, beliefs, values, expectations, and goals. Our perceptions of the world around us are culturally learned and mediated. People from different cultural backgrounds perceive the world differently. Scholars argue that there is no single universal reality and that many possible understandings of behaviors, interactions, or events are determined by social and cultural contexts.

Non-Latino therapists must be humble in their role as learners, not experts. They must assume a nonknowing stance. They do not have access to privileged information and cannot fully understand a person from another culture. They are obliged to learn the culture of the client from the perspective of that person and must be very respectful of the client's understandings and positions regarding his or her problem. The result is a collaboration between client and psychotherapist (Kleinman, 1980), not a one-up/one-down relationship in which the therapist dominates the dialogue to correct the client's faulty thinking or behavior. As Kleinman argues, the client's stated problem has to be the problem. One cannot correct faulty logic but rather initiate a dialogue to generate multiple possibilities in order to solve the problem.

Many writers in this area have emphatically pointed out the ubiquity of the influence of culture in evaluation and treatment. There is a real need in mental health care delivery to render services responsible to the client's cultural identity. The clinician must attempt, for example, to formally assess whether reports of unusual beliefs, such as belief in spirits, constitute psychopathology or a purely cultural perspective (Fabrega, 1995). Fabrega has drawn attention to the need to modify Axis II categories (personality disorders) as well as Axis IV (stressors) and Axis V (adaptive functioning) to render them appropriate in Latin American social settings.

Fabrega (1995) brings up a series of questions that the mental health practitioner, Spanish-speaking or not, needs to address. The first asks about the DSM categories of illness and if they should be modified to accommodate Latino realities. Second, do biological factors dominating establishment psychiatry override clinical complexity? Third, should the complexity of the migration/acculturation experience put it in a class by itself, especially in light of the complex social and psychological adjustments it engenders? Surely the case of Dora, hiding behind bushes and making her way north from Guatemala to the U.S.-Mexican border, is not the average emotional trauma of being fired from a job or losing a loved one. Thus, migratory experience may need to become a legitimate and authentic stressor in any mental health nosological system.

Fabrega (1995) also wonders about the benefits or deficits that accrue to Latinos who resort to indigenous healing traditions. Can we say that indigenous healing traditions can surpass establishment ones, even if the latter are rendered culturally sensitive? Fabrega relates how the growing Latino population in the United States encounters adaptive problems and challenges in a parent society and responds with both negative and positive adaptive changes. This, in turn, feeds back into molding science in a universalistic direction, permitting insight into the human condition despite ethnic membership. Fabrega, in this case, wants to use Latino realities to make establishment psychiatric conventions more representative and valid.

Curanderismo, the practice of folk healing, impacts rural and working-class populations of Mexico and other Latin American countries, as well as immigrants. *Curanderismo* blends a number of components, including herbal lore, supernatural elements, religion, and science along with Catholic dogma. As Mayers (1989) points out, newer social science literature on Latinos in the United States downplays the importance of *curanderismo,* even to the point of inconsequence. Jenkins and Karno (1992), for example, found that in Southern California, modern medicine has become the primary system for health and mental health services, with folk medicine an ancillary form of treatment mainly for minor health problems. However, since Mexican nationals continue to gravitate to established Mexican-American barrios, legally or illegally, it is important for the clinician to understand the worldview and structure of traditional folk healing. Sometimes folk medicine remains attractive to Latino immigrants because they become dissatisfied with some aspect of medical treatment that they receive from a physician or because they do not understand what is happening to them. An important role of the clinician is that of a teacher, to explain body processes and negotiate explanatory models with clients to help them understand depression, panic, etc.

From a practical point of view, there will be many times when the non-Latino therapist is obliged to use interpreters. The word alone is important to understand, as there is a difference between a translator (for textual materials) and an interpreter, who listens and presents the material in English.

USING INTERPRETERS

Interpreters are often used in health agencies and in private practice. When the psychotherapist is not bilingual and needs to employ an interpreter, there are some important dos and don'ts to consider. The interpreter and the client often come from different geographical areas and cultural backgrounds. Additionally, distorted and confusing material may intrude, which can be intensified in a psychiatric setting. If the patient is confused or disoriented, the interpreter has to pay attention to the communication pattern, which may be full of tangential, hallucinatory, and delusional material or other pathological manifestations of mental illness.

Vasquez and Javier (1991) have pointed out five common errors that interpreters make, which include omission, additions, condensation, substitution, and role exchange. Omission means that the interpreter completely or partially deletes a message sent by the speaker. Addition is the tendency to include information not expressed by the speaker. Simplifying and explaining is referred to as condensation, and replacing concepts is called substitution. Role exchange occurs when the interpreter takes over an interaction and replaces the interviewer's questions with his or her own, becoming the interviewer in the process.

Untrained interpreters make all these errors. They take shortcuts or use literary license, and it is not unusual to note their deficiency in the client's primary language. Often, interpreters may be ignorant of regional colloquialisms. For example, Maria was sent to me through her EAP supervisor for fighting with a Mexican-American supervisor who accused her of using foul language. The word that Maria used in Guatemalan Spanish meant inconsequential, while in Mexico the same word was a filthy curse. In Peru, by contrast, the word means a shack where groceries are sold. The human resources office was ready to fire this poor woman due to this misunderstanding.

Using support staff such as security guards and janitors who may have some bilingual knowledge is not recommended. Such individuals see this unwanted role as burdensome, as they are taken away from their jobs and have to put in extra time to finish their normal tasks. Thus, they are less concerned with the accuracy of interpretation and only want to get the interview done. I remember a Spanish-speaking nurse at a regional burn center where I worked who was forced into the role of interpreter at the death of a patient. She was very insensitive to the suffering of the relatives, and it was clear to any observer that her first priority was to get on with her own job. Many agencies pay bilingual staff an additional hourly bonus for their interpreting skills, when they properly recognize this as meriting extra recompense.

It is important to avoid serious misunderstandings that can have implications for hospitalizing a patient or which result in the administration of incorrect medication. First of all, the interpreter must be trained so that every word and all imagery from the client is communicated to the psychotherapist. I remember an often-repeated anecdote about a large Los Angeles hospital that had a number of Chinese clients. When an elderly Chinese woman was said to have psychotic symptoms, a file clerk was called in to help interpret (he had no special training, nor was his knowledge of Chinese ever evaluated by a supervisor fluent in the language). The woman described her anxiety metaphorically, stating that it was as if she had a dragon moving about in her stomach. The young interpreter said that the woman actually had a dragon in her stomach. The client was hospitalized unnecessarily and subsequent interactions between the clinician and the client were badly damaged.

We have all listened to a patient speaking in a foreign language who gives a long tirade, and the interpreter simply states that the woman is sad. It must be impressed upon the interpreter that no ambiguity is tolerated. In 1990-1991, I was in charge of a staff training activity in a large mental health hospital in Los Angeles, which included case presentations by staff who worked with monolingual, Spanish-speaking patients. On one occasion, a woman responded to the interviewer's questions in a barrage of Spanish. In my own evaluation of the client, it appeared to me that her speech was pressured, a clinical warning of the possibility that she suffered from a manic disorder. An excellent interpreter was present, who did a good job of capturing the client's remarks. However, since I was the only other person present who understood Spanish, the visiting clinicians were unable to ascertain if the patient's speech patterns indicated pressured speech. They would have been able to do so easily had the client been speaking English. I realized then how easy it would be to train a staff interpreter to recognize three types of Spanish speech patterns: a typical slow, normal, or excessively fast cadence and beat. This could be done using verbal samples and tape recordings until the professional interpreter could safely say that a particular client was speaking at a normal, slow, or accelerated pace, according to the standards previously developed. Needless to say, this would be very helpful in diagnosis, especially when psychopharmacological needs have to be factored in and correct diagnosis is crucial.

Psychotherapists must know and apply patterns of cultural etiquette in introducing themselves to the client and family. Minimal greetings in Spanish (hello, good afternoon, how are you, etc.) need to be mastered, even though the psychotherapist may not speak the language well. Indeed, Spanish is not a very difficult language for the English speaker to learn, since everything written is pronounced in a predictable way. There are only five vowel sounds to learn compared to the eighteen or so in English. The interpreter's chair must be placed behind the patient, not in a circle or next to the client. The therapeutic alliance must be established between the client and the psychotherapist, not between the client and the interpreter. If the patient has to turn around to speak to the interpreter rather than seeing the interpreter when facing the psychotherapist, it is likely that the patient will pay little attention to the interpreter.

It is unacceptable for the interpreter to be the patient's minor or adolescent child. Often, intimate details may be recounted. Hearing about family dysfunction, family secrets, sexual conflicts, etc., literally can stress a young child to the point of ulcers. To have a professional interpreter corps is clearly the optimum goal in an agency or clinic setting. If the psychotherapist uses a secretary or file clerk to interpret, he or she must be careful about Latin American social class differences because of the risk of *envidia* (envy) and prejudice due to gradients of skin color and social status differences. Once at a large medical center I observed a dark-skinned interpreter (supposedly professionally trained) incorrectly translate the doctor's comments into Spanish because she was envious of the fair hair and light skin color of the patient. The client was anxiously waiting to hear whether she needed an operation. On many occasions, I have been the second person present who understood Spanish when a so-called interpreter committed a major error. In forensic settings, this can be a great disservice to the client. Once I consulted with a lawyer who tried to help a neurologically disabled patient, Pedro, establish his competency to sue. I listened as a young man interpreted the lawyer's questions. Later, I took the lawyer aside to let him know that the young man who was the interpreter did not know the subjunctive tense in Spanish, a tense that deals with uncertainty and ambiguity. There was no way

that the lawyer *might* (subjective tense) establish the client's competency unless he could query the client using the full scope of the client's language to ensure correct communication.

Interpreters should have at least the equivalent of a high school
diploma, but some college or technical training is preferable. That the
individual had a long-deceased grandma or grandpa is just not sufficient. There is a real lack of standards today in the domain of interpreting, short of the criminal justice system, where at least in most states
there are court-established qualifying tests and standards. In most psychotherapy settings, there is no guarantee that an interpreter will do the
job correctly. Nothing should be taken for granted. A second opinion
or some independent evaluation of the interpreter's competence is
essential. When I applied for a position in a child guidance clinic during my training, a Panamanian woman interviewed me in Spanish, as
the director sat in. We spoke in Spanish for several minutes as part of
the interview. When I work with bilingual managed care case managers, we generally have at least one long conversation about the weather,
weekend activities, or even clinical information that is garnered infor-
mally by telephone to assess that the clinician indeed can speak the language adequately.

In a brilliant essay, Comas-Diaz (1992) argues that as the result of
the browning of America, a number of psychological values and
expectations will undergo major transformation in Euro-American
society. The independence of the client will be only one alternative and
other cultural values of interdependence will be seen as a mature
developmental response. There will be an externalization of coping
styles and a reliance on faith, prayer, and spirituality, in contrast with
the secular worldview of large numbers of psychotherapists. Even in
the rational-emotive therapy so useful with Latino immigrants, the
skeptical position that belief in God and spirituality are irrational needs
to be set aside. The client's religiosity should be respected when present. Of course, the therapist must be careful not to impose any particular form of spirituality on the client. In fact, shamanistic healing may
be on the rise as psychotherapy turns to explanatory models from
ethnocultural indigenous healing models. Even the infamous Oedipus
complex can be said to reflect Western thinking and psychology and
may have no place in the new multicultural psychotherapy.

Vargas and Koss-Chioino (1992) make a plea for culturally responsive therapy in which culture is actively integrated into psychotherapeutic interventions. These authors point out that there is not only one psychology. Rather, indigenous psychologies conceptualize individualism differently than the Euro-American model. A distinction is made between two types of individualism: self-contained and ensemble. Self-contained individualism is characterized by firm self-other boundaries, with an emphasis on personal control and an exclusionary concept of self. In contrast, an ensemble individualism is characterized by fluid self-other boundaries, field independence (versus field dependence), and an inclusive concept of the self. Cushman (1990), too, argues that there are only local theories about the self, and the bounded, masterful self is a deceit. In recent U.S. history, according to Cushman, there has been a deterioration of community, tradition, and shared meaning. We cannot deny the presence of cultural factors by emphasizing the structural aspects of self-psychology. Rather, we need to integrate cultural meaning and culturally relevant form and process into psychotherapy with ethnic minorities. An example that Vargas and Koss-Chioini (1992) give is the way that Puerto Rican and Mexican families groom females and often male children to remain at home until they marry.

In recent years, concepts of globalization have affected the Latino immigrant's integration into American society. In addition to racist attitudes and types of prejudice that Latinos face throughout the acculturation process, elements of the dominant majority culture have many effects on the Latino immigrant. These include how recently immigrants settled in the United States, the ethnicity and social organization of the community in which immigrants settle, their preimmigration experiences, and their personal adjustment prior to the full impact of the acculturation process. The non-Latino therapist must pay attention to the effects of acculturation—the way in which cultural change or interchange affects the ethnic group and how it may lose aspects of its cultural differences or may exaggerate aspects of its ethnic integrity (Vargas and Koss-Chioino, 1992).

In a challenging article, Bibeau (1997) writes that the world we live in is changing in a very unusual way. We are beginning to live at the interface of both our local world and a larger, global world where we become trapped between fidelity to our own cultural identity and the global community. Yet, we must assume a more flexible, pluralist frame of reference when we deal with the larger world. Many major changes have affected the quality of life globally in the last several decades, including economic disintegration, social disruptions, disordered urbanization, political repression, and huge migration, to name a few. The globalization associated with multinational enterprises, planetary economic markets, and interstate capital flows has impacted all levels of peoples and has internationalized youth cultures to cause a de facto multiculturalism. Every place in the world is very permeable to influences from elsewhere. The Latino rural peasant in Iquitos in the Peruvian tropical rain forest has better TV reception, with multiple channels due to a large satellite disk in that city, than I do in Southern California. The world system influences every nook and cranny in our lives.

The spread of modernity and general access to commodities creates problems for the psychotherapist—as fuzzy boundaries allow more and more people to share cultural patterns. Although people may be grounded in their local worlds, they participate in the global system. Individuals have both personal identity and relationships to multiple communities, to which many people belong simultaneously. This includes: (1) the culture of one's early socialization; (2) one's citizenship identity, where we attain civil rights, and (3) the social participation of a person in the host country where the person is transplanted. People have to reconstruct their identities when they have been separated from the original culture by immigration or exposure to foreign cultures.

Bibeau (1997) finds that cultural psychiatry deals with identity systems, such as language and symbols, which are threatened by the globalization process. In complex societies, Bibeau argues, what generates diversity and hierarchy is knowledge, not just capital. Class divisions are filtered through the distribution of knowledge. Society is becoming controlled by experts—professionals, intellectuals— persons of knowledge. Knowledge has replaced traditional wisdom of the past.

That non-Latinos should find themselves in a position to counsel Latino clients, given this situation, is by no means unusual. The expert, or the psychotherapist, in many cases, is called upon to proffer wisdom and recommendations that in the past would have been the province of elders, priests, and other community members.

The whole world has been Europeanized or Westernized—the result of unequal encounters between conquering Western nations and defeated, colonized peoples. We live in a time with ambiguous notions of authenticity. There is much resentment, often about who should be the representative voice of a given ethnic group or gender. The psychotherapist who takes the time to learn about the Latino community—its needs in the translocation and immigration process—has every right to enter the global arena. Mental health issues of the immigrant client are challenging, and work with this population can bring immense satisfaction to the practitioner.

If counselors originate from a sector of the larger society that has little familiarity with patterns of Latin American culture, they will probably be ineffective, especially if they hold strong stereotypes. Smart and Smart (1995), in turn, suggest that immigrants approach counselors with suspicion and mistrust, unsure if the counselors are genuinely interested in creating a therapeutic alliance. Counselors may have difficulties in excusing the hardships and pain that unjust social practices perpetuate. Counselors who have not previously worked with poverty issues may be overwhelmed by the many problems and needs of the clients. It may impose difficulties for them to understand Latino clients' lifestyles and their decisions and actions.

A client can easily feel brushed off by an uncaring and unresponsive system and experience the counselor's efforts as half-hearted. Anglo culture, in general, may appear to the Latino to be cold, uncaring, bureaucratic, and social distances generally separate the client and the counselor. The Latino male's macho attitude of independence may make him feel a sense of failure if he is unable to be a successful wage earner. To approach a counselor may make him appear weak or inadequate. Such feelings can keep him from seeking help to alleviate acculturation stress, and he may postpone or forgo treatment for physical, mental, or emotional problems.

The non-Latino counselor may see one of two responses to mental health problems that the client faces. On one hand, the client may rely heavily on propitiatory religious rituals instead of medical or psychotherapeutic intervention and attribute his life experiences to God's will. Such religious fatalism needs to be challenged in the therapeutic process rather than ignored. Liberal quotes from the Bible to illustrate a psychotherapeutic point can be very useful for such clients. Or the client may be overly compliant and bestow an exaggerated respect on the psychotherapist as a consequence of culturally based deference toward perceived authority figures. This can lead to the psychotherapist becoming overinvolved with the patient, and a stultifying dependence of the client. There is a real difference, as Comas, Diaz, and Griffith (1988) argue, between pathological defenses and adaptive coping as we try to understand the client.

While traditional psychotherapy posits the therapist as an expert who conceptualizes the case and/or the specific treatment plan, this approach is not always useful with multicultural clients. The therapist does not have access to privileged information and cannot ever fully understand another person. Rather, the therapist must make every effort to learn the culture of the client as the client sees it. The therapist has to ascertain not only the way that clients see themselves as similar to others within their culture, but also as unique in their beliefs, lifestyle, behavior, attribution of meanings, etc. Sue (1992) wisely suggests that the therapist who works with immigrant populations should allow for more than one answer to a problem and for more than one way to arrive at a solution. The therapist should always have a strong sense of curiosity about the client's story or problem. A priori assumptions about a client should, at best, be put on hold. Even a therapist who is sensitive or familiar with cultural concerns may be off-target. The therapist must not dominate the dialogue in an effort to correct the client's faulty thinking or behavior. Rather, therapist and client must mutually search for alternate ideas and expand the behavioral options that have emerged from a dialogue about a given issue. The therapist can use *dichos* or cultural proverbs rather than presenting new narratives. Latino immigrants basically want answers to their problems.

The psychotherapist can value the independence of the client but must also recognize the value of interdependence, which he or she should see as a desirable trait. As Comas-Diaz (1992) suggests, faith and prayer are not to be seen skeptically as some kind of deficiency in the client, but as an externalizing coping style. Nor will spiritual values be diminished—just the contrary. When faced with a religious client, I often ask if he or she has met with a minister or priest to discuss the issue in question. Comas-Diaz shows a healthy respect for ethnocultural indigenous models of healing. Calming teas, salves, prayers, etc., are well worth reaffirming if they do no harm.

Counseling techniques must be modified to match the specific culture of the client. Psychotherapists must be sensitive in working with persons of different racial and ethnic minority backgrounds (see Pedersen, 1991). Atkinson (1983) says that counselors assume the roles of advisor, advocate, and facilitator of indigenous support and healing systems, change agents as well as psychologists or counselors. They must quickly assess clients' level of acculturation so as to know how hard to push and what kind of psychoeducational role they will play in clients' lives, even if only briefly.

I have never regretted my intense interest in Latino mental health and hope that the insights I have been able to gain from this work can be incorporated into the psychotherapeutic practices of others throughout the United States, as needed. Multicultural perspectives can contribute to brief therapy, if the therapist is willing to take the time to learn about the cultural background and needs of the client.

Appendix A

Hypnotic Inductions
in English and Spanish

SUGGESTIONS AND METAPHORS
FOR POST-TRAUMATIC STRESS DISORDER
AND PAIN CONTROL
(ENGLISH TRANSLATION)

Dialogue Prior to Hypnotic Induction

I want to explain just what happens to you now that you have experienced an accident or burn trauma [substitute exact type of trauma or accident experienced by patient]. You see, the body responds in a very special way after you experience a trauma like the one you have just had. This trauma is felt in the body, especially in the muscle system.

You know, your blood flows through your veins and arteries very much like the irrigation canals you remember from your home country. That is, when we use very high-powered microscopes, we see that the arteries and veins have walls, very small so that the eye can't see them, but these walls are made up of muscles. The whole thing is like an irrigation canal you know so well in Mexico, you know, when the mud falls into the canal, the water cannot flow to irrigate the plants and crops. In this way, when you have an accident [trauma], the muscles of the walls of your arteries and veins get narrower and narrower until your blood doesn't flow as much and as quickly as it should. Just like the mud in the irrigation canal falling into the water, your arteries and veins get smaller and your hands get cold, and you get tense; it is like a little tiger ready to attack. That is the startle effect you feel very often.

Well, there are special exercises that I am going to teach you which will help you to communicate with your muscles. It appears to be a lie, but indeed it is true, that we can indeed control our own muscles, and we can make these irrigation canals in our body open, and we can allow our blood to flow normally the way it should. So, I will sit here in this chair, and you will sit over there and close your eyes and simply follow the words that I say. When I am finished, I will say to you, "Open your eyes." Do you understand? OK, let's begin.

Induction

Pay attention to your breathing. . . . Breathe in slowly, breathe out slowly, listen to the sound of my voice and try not to sleep, and with each breath that you take, feel yourself becoming more and more relaxed, more and more relaxed, calm, and tranquil.

Feel fresh energy passing through your body; move that energy, little by little, through your body, from the top of your head, passing your forehead, your cheeks; feel your jaw relaxing, your mouth opening a little bit, as that energy passes to your shoulders. Take ten seconds and feel that cool energy passing through your body, from the top of your head to your shoulders. Begin now, one, two, three, four, more and more relaxed, calm and tranquil, five, six, seven, more and more relaxed, calm and tranquil, eight, nine, and ten.

Now, feel that cool energy passing through your body. Move it little by little, inside your body, from the shoulders, passing through your chest, through your back, to your waist. Take ten seconds to feel that fresh energy passing through your body. Move it little by little, into your body, from the shoulders to the waist. Begin now, one, two, three, more and more relaxed, more and more relaxed, calm and tranquil, four, five, six, very calm, seven, eight, nine, and ten, the most relaxed feeling that you have ever felt.

Now, feel the fresh energy passing through your body. Move it little by little into your body, from the shoulders, passing your arm, passing your elbow, passing your wrist, to the tips of your fingers. Take ten seconds to feel the fresh energy passing through your body. Move it little by little into your body, from the shoulders to the tips of your fingers. Begin now. One, two, three, more and more relaxed, calm and tranquil, four, five, and six, more and more relaxed, calm and tranquil, seven, eight, nine, and ten, the most relaxed feeling that you have ever felt, as if you were floating on top of a pretty white cloud in a blue sky, so calm, so tranquil.

Now, feel the fresh energy pass into your body. Move it little by little into your body, from the waist, past your thighs, past your knees to your feet. Take ten seconds to feel the fresh energy pass through your body. Move it little by little into your body, from the waist to the feet. Begin now. One, two, three, calm and tranquil, four, five, six, more and more relaxed, calm and tranquil, seven, eight, nine, and ten, the most relaxed feeling you have ever felt.

Now, imagine that you are standing by the seashore. You feel very relaxed, calm, very happy, at ease. Feel the breeze caress your face, smell the fresh air, feel the cool sand on your feet—more and more relaxed, more and more relaxed, calm and tranquil.

Now imagine that you are in a beautiful pine forest. It is a spring day. Smell the fresh air, listen to the sound of the birds, see the flowers in all their colors. You feel very good, tranquil, calm, very calm, very tranquil.

If There Are Problems in Sleeping

Now, imagine that you are in your house. It is nighttime; you are sleeping in your bed. Imagine you are sleeping well, all night long, having happy dreams, pretty dreams, tranquil dreams, without waking up, breathing peacefully all night long. You feel very well, calm, tranquil, very relaxed.

If There Are Problems of Pain

Now, imagine that you have a green pitcher of ice water, very cold. Put your right hand inside the pitcher, and feel the cold passing to that right hand, until it is very numb, so that you don't feel it at all. Now, place that right hand on whatever part of your body is bothering you, and little by little, feel that coldness pass to your body. You feel very good, calm and tranquil, very relaxed.

If There Are Problems with Body Image
After an Accident or Injury

Imagine that you are in your house, in front of your mirror. How handsome (pretty) you are. You feel very tranquil. Your hand (or whatever part of the body that is affected) is fine. Imagine that your are in your house, in front of your mirror, how handsome you are, how tranquil you feel. You are like the eagle, king of the birds, king of all his dominion. Whenever you want, wherever you are, with the tape or without the tape, you know how to calm yourself. Simply close your eyes, pay attention to your breathing, and little by little, feel that fresh energy pass into your body, little by little. You are like the king eagle, king of all your dominion, because you know how to calm yourself. You know how to relax.

To Realert the Client

Now, I am going to count from one to ten. Imagine that you are walking up a pretty staircase, and with each number that I say, feel that you are walking up the staircase. You feel more and more alert with each step, very awake, one, two, three, more and more alert, very happy, four, five, six, very, very alert, more and more awake, seven, eight, nine, and ten. Open your eyes.

SPANISH TRANSLATION

Diálogo Antes de la Inducción

Quiero explicarle exactamente lo que le pasa ahora que Vd. ha experimentado un acidente o quemadura [substituya el tipo exacto de trauma o acidente experimentado por el paciente]. Mire, el cuerpo responde al accidente de una manera especial como aquello que recientemente ha tenido Vd. Este trauma se siente en el cuerpo, especialmente en el sistema muscular.

Sabe, la sangre corre por sus venas y arterias tal como en los canales de irrigacíon que Vd. recuerda de su tierra. Es decir, cuando utilizamos un microscopio de alto poder, vemos que las paredes de las arterias y las venas son muy pequenas que el ojo no puede verlas, pero estas paredes estan hechas de músculos. Todo esto es como un canal de irrigacion que Vd. conoce tan bien en Mexico, Vd. sabe, cuando el barro cae dentro del canal, el agua no puede correr para irrigar a las plantas y las cosechas. De igual manera, cuando Vd. se acidenta, los músculos de las arterias y las venas se obstruyen de tal manera que su sangre no corre libremente. Justo, como el barro en el canal de irrigacion que cae al agua, igualmente sus arterias y sus venas se estrechan y sus manos se enfrian y Vd. se pone tenso. Es como un tigrillo listo para saltar en ataque. Esto es el susto que Vd. siente muy frecuentamente.

Ahora bien, hay ejercicios especiales que voy a enseñarle que le ayudarán a comunicarse con sus músculos. Parece mentira, pero es la verdad, podemos controlar a nuestros propios músculos y podemos hacer que estos canales de irrigacíon en nuestro cuerpo se abran y podemos permitir que nuestra sangre corra normalmente. Pues, voy a sentarme aqui en la silla, y Vd. se sienta alli, y cierre los ojos y simplemente escuche a las palabras que yo digo. Cuando termino, voy a decirle, "abra los ojos." Comprende Vd.? Bien, empezamos.

Inducción en Espánol

Preste atencíon a la respiracíon. . . . Aspire Vd. lentamente . . . expire Vd. lentamente, escucha el sonido de mi voz y procure no dormir . . . y con cada respiracion, se va sentir mas y mas relajado, mas y mas relajado, calmo y tranquilo.

Siente la energia que es fresca, va a pasar por su cuerpo. . . . Tiene que moverla poco a poco, dentro su cuerpo . . . desde la corona de la cabeza, pasando la frente, pasando las mejillas. . . . La mandíbula relajada, la boca abre un poco . . . pasando el cuello hasta los hombros. Tome diez segundos para sentir la energia va a pasar por su cuerpo, desde la corona de la cabeza hasta los hombros. Empezamos ahora. Uno, dos, tres, cuatro, mas y mas relajado, calmo y tranquilo, cinco, seis, siete, mas y mas relajado, calmo y tranquilo, ocho, nueve, y diez.

Ahora siente la energia que es fresca, va a pasar por su cuerpo. Tiene que môverla poco a poco, dentro su cuerpo, desde los hombros, pasando el pecho, pasando la espalda hasta la cintura. Tome diez segundos para sentir la energia que es fresca, va a pasar por su cuerpo. Tiene que moverla poco a poco, dentro su cuerpo . . . desde los hombros, hasta la cintura. Empezamos ahora, uno, dos, tres, mas y mas relajado, mas y mas relajado, calmo y tran- quillo, cuatro, cinco, seis, bien calmo, siete, ocho, nueve, diez, el mas relajado que nunca sentia.

Ahora, siente la energia que es fresca, va a pasar por su cuerpo. Tiene que moverla poco a poco, dentro su cuerpo, desde los hombros, pasando el brazo, pasando el codo, pasando la muñeca, hasta las yemas de los dedos. Tome diez segundos para sentir la energia que es fresca, va a pasar por el cuerpo, tiene que moverla poco a poco, dentro su cuerpo, desde los hombros, hasta las yemas de los dedos. Empezamos ahora, uno, dos, tres, mas y mas relajado, calmo y tranquilo, cuatro, cinco, seis, mas y mas relajado, calmo y tranquilo, siete, ocho, nueve, y diez, el mas relajado que nunca sentia, si fuera flotando encima de una nube bonita, blanca en un cielo azul, tan calmo, tan tranquilo.

Ahora, siente la energia que es fresca, va pasar por su cuerpo. Tiene que môverla poco a poco, dentro su cuerpo, desde la cintura, pasando los muslos, pasando las rodillas, hasta los pies. Tome diez segundos para sentir la energia que es fresca, va a pasar por su cuerpo. Tiene que moverla poco a poco, dentro su cuerpo, desde la cintura hasta los pies. Empezamos ahora, uno, dos, tres, calmo y tranquilo, cuatro, cinco, seis, mas y mas relajado, calmo y tranquilo, siete, ocho, nueve, y diez, el mas relajado que nunca sentia.

Ahora, imagine Vd. que esta parado por la orilla del mar. Vd. siente relajado, calmo, bien a gusto, alegre. Siente la brisa cariciar en su cara, huela el aire fresco, siente la arena fresca en sus pies descalzos, mas y mas relajado, mas y mas relajado, calmo y tranquilo.

Ahora, imagine Vd. que esta en un bosque bonito, de pinos. Es un dia de la primavera. Huela el aire fresca, escucha el sonido de los pájaros, vea las flores de todos colores. Vd. siente muy bien, tranquilo, calmo, bien calmo, bien tranquilo.

Si Hay Problema Con el Dormir

Ahora, imagine Vd. que esta en su casa. Es noche, está dormiendo en su cama. Imagine que está dormiendo bien, toda la noche, teniendo suenos alegres, bonitos, tranquilos, sin despertarse, respirando con tranquilidad, toda la noche. Vd. siente muy bien, calmo, tranquilo, bien relajado.

Si Hay Problemas de Dolor en el Cuerpo

Ahora, imagine Vd. que tiene un jarro verde de agua helada, bien helada. Ponga Vd. la mano derecha dentro el jarro, y siente que el frio va pasando a la mano derecho, hasta que esta entumecida bien, que no la siente. Ahora, tome la mano derecha a donde en su cuerpo esta molestando, y poco a poco siente la frialdad pasa al cuerpo. Vd. siente muy bien, calmo y tranquilo, bien relajado.

Si Hay Problemas de Desgusto del Cuerpo
Despues del Acidente, Injurio, etc.

Imagine que está en su casa, frente a su espejo. Que lindo (guapo) está, tranquilo, su mano está bien, esta linda, imagine que está en su casa, frente su espejo, que linda esta, que bonita, tranquila.

Vd. es como el rey águila, rey do todo su dominio. Cuando quiere, donde sea, con la cinta o sin al cinta, Vd. sabe calmarse. Vd. simplemente tiene que cerrar los ojos, hacer caso a la respiracíon, y poco a poco, siente la energia que es fresca, va a pasar pos su cuerpo, poco a poco. Vd. es como el rey águila, rey de todo su dominio, porque Vd. sabe calmarse, sabe relajarse.

Para Despertarle al Cliente

Ahora, voy a contar de uno a diez. Imagine que está subiendo una escalera bonita, y con cada numero que digo, siente que esta subiendo la escalera, y se siente mas y mas alerto con cada peldaño, muy despierto, uno, dos, tres, mas y mas alerto, bien a gusto va, cuatro, cinco, seis, mas y mas alerto, mas despierto, siete, ocho, nueve, y diez. Abre los ojos!

Appendix B

Tests, Scales, and Resources Available in Spanish

PARENTING EDUCATION

Russell Barkley and Christine M. Benton (1997). *Niños desafiantes: Materiales de evaluacion y folletos para los padres.* Trans. Jose Banermeister. New York: Guilford Press.

"Daily duties," Sun Sales, Inc. P.O. Box 1315, Cardiff, CA 92007 (760-431-7209) (see p. 159).

Lupita Montoya and Kerby T. Alva, *Manual para los padres: Version español.* Center for the Improvement of Child Caring, Studio City, CA.

Padres eficaces con entrenamiento sistemático. (Spanish edition of STEP—see Dinkemayer, McKay, and Dinkmayer, in references). AGS, 4201 Woodland Road, P.O. Box 99, Circle Pines, MN 55014-1796.

ATTENTION DEFICIT AND HYPERACTIVITY DISORDER RESOURCES

Home Scales in Spanish: Stephen B. McCarney (1994). "Formulario de evaluacion en version domestica." Hawthorne Educational Services, 800 Gray Oak Drive, Columbia, MO 65201 (1-800-542-1673).

Stephen B. McCarney and Angela Marie Bauer (1994). *The parent's guide to attention deficit disorders.* Columbia, MO: Hawthorne Educational Services, Inc.

Vineland Adaptive Behavior Scales (in Spanish). AGS, 4201 Woodland Road, P.O. Box 99, Circle Pines, MN 55014-1796.

BOOK RESOURCES

Jess Araujo (1998). *La ley y sus derechos.* 1324 N. Broadway, Santa Ana, CA 92706 (714-835-6990).

Kurt F. Geisinger, ed. (1992). *Psychological testing of Hispanics.* Washington, DC: American Psychological Association.

Steven M. Kaplan (1995). *Wiley's English-Spanish dictionary of psychology and psychiatry.* New York: John Wiley and Sons.

DAILY DUTIES

Learn Good Habits and Responsibility, Do Your Duty. Use This Daily List and Check all Completed Duties

DAILY DUTIES

MY WORK WAS THIS WEEK

Name:

TAKE CARE OF MYSELF	S	M	T	W	T	F	S
Shower or Bath							
Brush My Teeth							
Other							

TAKE CARE OF MY ROOM	S	M	T	W	T	F	S
Put My Things Away & Make My Bed							
Put My Clothes Away							
Other							

FAMILY DUTIES	S	M	T	W	T	F	S
Clean Up My Mess							
Take Out The Trash & Help With The Dishes							
Feed My Pet							
Outside Chores							
Other							

SCHOOL DUTIES	S	M	T	W	T	F	S
Finish My Homework							
Did I Participate In Class							
Did I Learn Something New							
Other							

The Special Goal I'm Working Toward This Week Is:

GREAT JOB!

YOU'RE THE BEST!

WAY TO GO!

THANKS FOR YOUR HELP!

ASSERTIVENESS TRAINING

TABLE 1a. A Comparison of Passive, Assertive, and Aggressive Communication and the Consequences of Each

	When My Communication Is Passive I . . .	When My Communication Is Assertive I . . .	When My Communication Is Aggressive I . . .
Characteristics of the behavior	Ignore, do not express my own rights, needs, desires	Express and assert my own rights, needs, desires	Express my own rights at expense of others
	Permit others to infringe on my rights	Stand up for legitimate rights in a way that rights of others are not violated	Display inappropriate outbursts or hostile overreaction; Intend to humiliate, to "get even," to put the other down
	Am emotionally dishonest, indirect, inhibited, manipulative	Am emotionally honest, direct, expressive	Emotionally honest, direct, expressive at other's expense
	Self-denying	Am self-enhancing, persistent	Am self-enhancing
	Allow others to choose for me	Choose for myself	Choose for others
My feelings when I engage in this behavior	Feel hurt, anxious, disappointed in myself at the time and possibly angry later	Am confident, self-respecting, feel good about myself at the time and later	Am angry then righteous, superior, depreciatory at the time, possibly guilty later
Outcome	Do not achieve desired goal(s)	May achieve desired goal(s)	Achieve desired goal(s) by hurting others
Payoff	Avoid unpleasant and risky situations, avoid conflict, sensing confrontation; don't get needs met; Accumulate anger; Feel nonvalued	Feel good; am valued by myself and others; Feel better about myself; improve self-confidence; have my needs met; my relationships are freer, more honest	Saving up anger, resentment to justify a blow-up, an emotional outburst, "to get even, get back at"
	Passive Behavior	Assertive Behavior	Aggressive Behavior
Other people's feelings about themselves when I engage in this behavior	Guilty, superior, or angry	Valued, respected	Hurt, humiliated
Other people's feelings about me when I engage in this behavior	Irritated, pity, disgusted	Generally respectful	Angry, vengeful

Source: From *Your Perfect Right: A Guide to Assertive Living* (Seventh Edition). © 1995 by Robert E. Alberti and Michael L. Emmons. Reproduced by permission of Impact Publishers, Inc., PO Box 6016, Atascadero, CA 93423. Further reproduction prohibited.

TABLE 1b. Summary of Communication Behaviors

	PASSIVE	ASSERTIVE	AGGRESSIVE
I. VERBAL			
I speak....	Apologetic words	My wants	Loaded words
	Veiled meanings	Honest statement of feelings	Accusations
	Hedging: failure to come to point	Objective words	Descriptive, subjective terms
	Rambling, disconnected	Direct statements that say what I mean	Imperious, superior words
	Not saying what I really mean	"I" messages	"You" messages
	"I mean," "You know"		
II. NON-VERBAL			
A. Generally, I use ...	Actions instead of speaking, hoping someone will guess what I want	Display attentive listening behavior	Exaggerated show of strength
	Looking as if I don't mean what I say	General assured manner, communication, caring, and strength	Flippant, sarcastic style
B. Specific			
1. My voice is ...	Weak, hesitant, soft, sometimes wavering	Firm, warm, well-modulated, relaxed	Tense, shrill, loud, shaky, cold, "deadly quiet"; demanding, superior, authoritative
2. My eyes are ...	Averted, downcast, teary, pleading	Open, frank, direct	Expressionless; narrowed; cold; staring; not really "seeing" you
3. Other			
a. My stance is ...	Leaning for support; twisted	Well-balanced; straight-on; at ease	Hands on hips; feet apart
b. My posture is ...	Stooped, "shrunken"; sagging; excessive head nodding	Facing, erect, relaxed	Stiff and rigid, rude
c. My hands are	Fidgety, fluttery, clammy	Relaxed, warm, smooth motions	Clenched; abrupt gesture; finger-pointing; fist pounding
d. My feet are ...	Shuffling, making restless motions: tucked under chair; toed-in: swinging back and forth	Relaxed, comfortable position	Tapping: firmly planted

159

TABLE 1c. Comunicación Pasiva, Apropriada, y Agresiva

	Cuando mi comunicación es pasivo, yo . . .	Cuando mi comunicación es asertivo, yo . . .	Cuando mi comunicación es agresivo, yo . . .
Caracteristicas del comportamiento	No expreso mis propios derechos, necesidades o deseos Soy deshonesto emocionalmente, indirecto, inhibido, manipulativo, permito que lo demas gente elija por mi	Expreso y afirmo mis derechos, necesidades y deseos Exijo mis derechos legitimos de tal manera que no violan los derechos de los demas Soy honesto emocionalmente directo y expresivo Soy persistente, elijo por mi-mismo	Expreso mis propios derechos en vez de aquellos de lo demas gente Muestro sobre-reacciones hostiles o inapropriadas; quiero humiliar o vengarme de lo demas Soy honesto directo, expresivo por lo que sufre lo demas gente; elijo por lo demas gente
Mis emociones cuando hago tal comportamiento	Me siento ansioso, triste o tal ez enojado contra mi-mismo mas tarde	Me respeto a mi-mismo y me siento a gusto tanto ahore como mas tarde	Siento coraje, después me siento superior, a veces culpable mas tarde
Efectos	No logro mis metas deseados	Puedo lograr mis metas deseados	Logro mis deseos pero causo sufrimiento a otros
Beneficios	Evito situaciones arriesgadas e incómodas, evito confrontacion, pero mis necesidades no son satisfechas; el coraje se acumula, no tengo sentido de estimacion propia	Me siento bien, yo me auto-valorizo, me siento mejor acerca de mi-mismo, aumento mi Auto-confianza, mis deseos estan satisfechos, mis relaciones con la gente son mejores y mas honestas	Acumulo el coraje y resentimientos para justificar un momento desagradable—lucho para lograr venganza

TABLE 1d. Sumario de Comunicación y Comportamiento

	Comportamiento Pasivo	Comportamiento Apropriado	Comportamiento Agresivo
Cuáles son los sentimientos del otro hacia mí cuando hago este comportamiento?	Culpable, superior o enojado	Valorizado, respetado	Triste, humiliación
Cuáles son los sentimientos del otro hacia mí cuando hago este comportamiento?	Irritable, desgusto	Generalmente respetuoso	Venganza, coraje
Verbal: Yo hablo	Palabras con excusas, con sentimientos escondidos, indirectas, descontinuadas, no digo lo que verdaderamente quiero decir	Expreso mis anhelos, hago afirmaciones honestas de mis sentimientos; palabras objetivas, frases directas que dicen lo que quiero decir Mensajes del "yo"	Palabras que cuasan luchas acusaciones, términos subjetivos palabras de superioridad/inferioridad, mensajes sobre "Vd. o tu"
No-verbal	Utilizo acciones en vez de hablar; espero que alguien adivina lo que quiero; parece que no quiero lo que digo; el tono de mi voz es hesitante, dulce, a veces no fuerte; mis ojos miran abajo, tienen lágrimas; mi postura es achicada, mis manos estan mojadas; mis pies se mueven mucho	Yo muestro atención; mi manera es muy segura; muestra comunicación, cuidado, y fuerza El tono de mi voz es firme, bien mdulado, relajada Mis ojos estan abiertos, directos Mi postura esta bien balancead, relajada, erecta; mis manos estan calientes, relajadas, mis pies estan en posicion comoda	Muestro una fuerza exagerada utilizo un estilo sarcástico el tono de mi voz es tenso, fuerte, fria, superior, autoretativo Mis ojos no tienen expresion, fríos, no ven a la otra persona Mi postura muestra los pies aparte, estoy rigido, brusco

161

RATIONAL-EMOTIVE THERAPY TEST
OF IRRATIONAL THINKING

TABLE 2a. Personality Data Form

Instructions: Read each of the following items and circle after each one the word STRONGLY, MODERATELY, or WEAKLY to indicate how much you believe in the statement described in the item. Thus, if you strongly believe that it is awful to make a mistake when people are watching, circle the word STRONGLY in item 1; and if you weakly believe that it is intolerable to be disapproved by others, circle the word WEAKLY in item 2. DO NOT SKIP ANY ITEMS. Be as honest as you possibly can be.

Acceptance

1. I believe that it is awful to make a mistake when other people are watching.   STRONGLY   MODERATELY   WEAKLY

2. I believe that it is intolerable to be disapproved of by others.   STRONGLY   MODERATELY   WEAKLY

3. I believe that it is awful for people to know certain undesirable things about one's family or one's background.   STRONGLY   MODERATELY   WEAKLY

4. I believe that it is shameful to be looked down upon by people for having less than they have.   STRONGLY   MODERATELY   WEAKLY

5. I believe that it is horrible to be the center of attention of others who may be highly critical.   STRONGLY   MODERATELY   WEAKLY

6. I believe it is terribly painful when one is criticized by a person one respects.   STRONGLY   MODERATELY   WEAKLY

7. I believe that it is awful to have people disapprove of the way one looks or dresses.   STRONGLY   MODERATELY   WEAKLY

8. I believe that it is very embarrassing if people discover what one really is like.   STRONGLY   MODERATELY   WEAKLY

9. I believe that it is awful to be alone.   STRONGLY   MODERATELY   WEAKLY

10. I believe that it is horrible if one does not have the love or approval of certain special people who are important to me.   STRONGLY   MODERATELY   WEAKLY

11. I believe that one must have others on whom one can always depend for help.   STRONGLY   MODERATELY   WEAKLY

Frustration

12. I believe that it is intolerable to have things go along slowly and not be settled quickly.   STRONGLY   MODERATELY   WEAKLY

13. I believe that it is too hard to get down to work at things it often would be better for one to do.   STRONGLY   MODERATELY   WEAKLY

14. I believe that it is terrible that life is so full of inconveniences and frustrations.   STRONGLY   MODERATELY   WEAKLY

15. I believe that people who keep one waiting frequently are pretty worthless and deserve to be boycotted.   STRONGLY   MODERATELY   WEAKLY

16. I believe that it is terrible if one lacks desirable traits that other people possess.   STRONGLY   MODERATELY   WEAKLY

17. I believe that it is intolerable when other people do not do one's bidding or give one what one wants.   STRONGLY   MODERATELY   WEAKLY

18. I believe that some people are unbearably stupid or nasty and that one must get them to change.   STRONGLY   MODERATELY   WEAKLY

19. I believe that it is too hard for one to accept serious responsibility.   STRONGLY   MODERATELY   WEAKLY

20. I believe that it is dreadful that one cannot get what one wants without making a real effort to get it.   STRONGLY   MODERATELY   WEAKLY

21. I believe that things are too rough in this world and that therefore it is legitimate for one to feel sorry for oneself.   STRONGLY   MODERATELY   WEAKLY

22. I believe that it is too hard to persist at many of the things one starts, especially when the going gets rough.   STRONGLY   MODERATELY   WEAKLY

23. I believe that it is terrible that life is so unexciting and boring.   STRONGLY   MODERATELY   WEAKLY

24. I believe that it is awful for one to have to discipline oneself.   STRONGLY   MODERATELY   WEAKLY

Injustice

25. I believe that people who do wrong things should suffer strong revenge for their acts.   STRONGLY   MODERATELY   WEAKLY

26. I believe that wrongdoers and immoral people should be severely condemned.   STRONGLY   MODERATELY   WEAKLY

27. I believe that people who commit unjust acts are bastards and that they should be severely punished.   STRONGLY   MODERATELY   WEAKLY

Achievement

28. I believe that it is horrible for one to perform poorly.   STRONGLY   MODERATELY   WEAKLY

29. I believe that it is awful if one fails at important things.   STRONGLY   MODERATELY   WEAKLY

30. I believe that it is terrible for one to make a mistake when one has to make important decisions.   STRONGLY   MODERATELY   WEAKLY

31. I believe that it is terrifying for one to take risks or to try new things.   .   STRONGLY   MODERATELY   WEAKLY

Worth

32. I believe that some of one's thoughts or actions are unforgivable.   STRONGLY   MODERATELY   WEAKLY

33. I believe that if one keeps failing at things one is a pretty worthless person.   STRONGLY   MODERATELY   WEAKLY

34. I believe that killing oneself is preferable to a miserable life of failure.   STRONGLY   MODERATELY   WEAKLY

35. I believe that things are so ghastly that one cannot help feeling like crying much of the time.   STRONGLY   MODERATELY   WEAKLY

36. I believe that it is frightfully hard for one to stand up for oneself and not give in too easily to others.   STRONGLY   MODERATELY   WEAKLY

37. I believe that when one has shown poor personality traits for a long time, it is hopeless for one to change.	STRONGLY	MODERATELY	WEAKLY
38. I believe that if one does not usually see things clearly and act well on them one is hopelessly stupid.	STRONGLY	MODERATELY	WEAKLY
39. I believe that it is awful to have no good meaning or purpose in life.	STRONGLY	MODERATELY	WEAKLY

Control

40. I believe that one cannot enjoy oneself today because of one's early life.	STRONGLY	MODERATELY	WEAKLY
41. I believe that if one kept failing at important things in the past, one must inevitably keep failing in the future.	STRONGLY	MODERATELY	WEAKLY
42. I believe that once one's parents train one to act and feel in certain ways, there is little one can do to act or feel better.	STRONGLY	MODERATELY	WEAKLY
43. I believe that strong emotions like anxiety and rage are caused by external conditions and events and that one has little or no control over them.	STRONGLY	MODERATELY	WEAKLY

Certainty

44. I believe it would be terrible if there were no higher being or purpose on which to rely.	STRONGLY	MODERATELY	WEAKLY
45. I believe that if one does not keep doing certain things over and over again something bad will happen if I stop.	STRONGLY	MODERATELY	WEAKLY
46. I believe that things must be in good order for one to be comfortable.	STRONGLY	MODERATELY	WEAKLY

Catastrophizing

47. I believe that it is awful if one's future is not guaranteed.	STRONGLY	MODERATELY	WEAKLY
48. I believe that it is frightening that there are no guarantees that accidents and serious illness will not occur.	STRONGLY	MODERATELY	WEAKLY
49. I believe that it is terrifying for one to go to new places or meet a new group of people.	STRONGLY	MODERATELY	WEAKLY
50. I believe that it is ghastly for one to be faced with the possibility of dying.	STRONGLY	MODERATELY	WEAKLY

TABLE 2b. Terapia Racional-Emotiva Evaluacion Personal

	Fuertamente	Moderadamente	Debilmente
Ser aceptado			
1. Creo que es desastrozo hacer un error cuando me mira lo demas gente.	F	M	D
2. Creo que es intolerable ser disaprobado por lo demas gente.	F	M	D
3. Creo que es desastrozo cuando la gente conoce alguna informacíon indeseable sobre mi familia o mi formacíon.	F	M	D
4. Creo que me mortifico si me desprecia la gente porque tengo menos bienes que ellos.	F	M	D
5. Creo que es horrible ser el centro de atencíon de lo demas gente quien puede ser criticona.	F	M	D
6. Creo que es terriblemente doloroso cuando me critica una persona hacia quien tengo mucho respeto.	F	M	D
7. Creo que es desastrozo cuando la gente desaprueba de la manera en que uno parece o se viste.	F	M	D
8. Creo que me es verguensoso si la gente descubre como soy verdaderamente.	F	M	D
9. Creo que es terrible ser solo.	F	M	D
10. Creo que es horrible si uno no tiene el amor o aprobacion de cierta gente especial, quien para mi es importante.	F	M	D
11. Creo que uno debe tener otra gente con la quien se puede contar.	F	M	D
Frustracion			
12. Creo que es intolerable que las cosas andan lentamente y que no se arreglan rápidamente.	F	M	D
13. Creo que es demasiado dificil empezar trabajar unos asuntos importantes y necesarios.	F	M	D
14. Creo que es terrible que la vida está llena de inconvenientes y frustraciones.	F	M	D
15. Creo que la gente quienes nos hacen esperar frecuentamente son sin valor alguna y merece ser boicoteada.	F	M	D
16. Creo que es terrible si nos faltan rasgos deseables que tienen otra gente.	F	M	D
17. Creo que es intolerable cuando otra gente no cumple con lo que yo quiero y no me dan lo que quiero.	F	M	D
18. Creo que alguna gente es terriblemente estúpida o mala y que hay que hacerle cambiar.	F	M	D
19. Creo que es demasiado difícil aceptar una responsabilidad seria.	F	M	D

20. Creo que es terrible que uno no puede lograr lo que uno quiere sin hacer un verdadero esfuerzo para obtenirlo.   F   M   D

21. Creo que las cosas son muy difíciles en este mundo y pues es legítimo para sentirse lástima hacia si-mismo.   F   M   D

22. Creo que es demasiado difícil persistir en las cosas que uno empieza especialmente cuando el camino llega a ser difícil.   F   M   D

23. Creo que es terrible que la vida no es tan excitante y que me aburro.   F   M   D

24. Creo que es desastrozo que hay que disciplinarse en la vida.   F   M   D

Injusticia

25. Creo que la gente que se comporta mal debe sufrir fuerte retribucíon por sus actos.   F   M   D

26. Creo que los malos y la gente inmoral deben ser severamente condemnados.   F   M   D

27. Creo que la gente quien comete actos injustos es una persona sin conciencia y que debe ser castigada severamente.   F   M   D

Alcances

28. Creo que es horrible que uno se actua malo.   F   M   D

29. Creo que es desastrozo si uno failla en las cosas importantes.   F   M   D

30. Creo que es terrible hacer un error cuando hay que hacer decisiones importantes.   F   M   D

31 Creo que es horroroso cuando hay que tomar un riesgo o intentar unas cosas nuevas.   F   M   D

Auto-valorizacion

32. Creo que algo de mis pensamientos o acciones no se puede perdonar.   F   M   D

33. Creo que si uno sigue faillando en las cosas uno es una persona bastante sin valor.   F   M   D

34. Creo que matarse es preferible a una vida miserable.   F   M   D

35. Creo que las cosas son tan terribles que no puedo evitar llorar la gran mayoria de tiempo.   F   M   D

36. Creo que es bastante difícil defenderme y no entregarme facilmente a los demás.   F   M   D

37. Creo que cuando se muestra mal genio durante mucho tiempo, es imposible que uno cambie.   F   M   D

38. Creo que si no se ve las cosas claramente y actua bien, entonces uno parece ser estúpido.   F   M   D

39. Creo que es desatrozo que la vida no signifique nada o que uno no tiene meta en la vida.   F   M   D

Control

40. Creo que no se puede gozar de la vida ahora: por razon de nuestras experiencias anteriores. F M D

41. Creo que si uno siempre ha faillado en el pasado, inevitablemente faillará en el futuro. F M D

42. Creo que una vez que sus padres le enseñan actuar y sentir en cierta manera, hay poco que se puede hacer por actuar o sentirse mejor. F M D

43. Creo que las fuertes emociones tal como la ansiedad o el coraje estan causado por las condiciones y los eventos externas, de los cuales uno tiene muy poco control. F M D

Certeza

44. Creo que será terrible que no haya fin y propósito, o un ser suprema en que dependerse. F M D

45. Creo que si yo no deja de repetir ciertos actos rituales, vez tras vez, algo malo me pasará. (ex.: lavar los manos con repeticion) F M D

46. Creo que las cosas tienen que estar en buen orden para que me siento cómodo. F M D

Castástrofe

47. Creo que es desastrozo si mi futuro no está asegurado. F M D

48. Me da terror que faltan garantias que los acidentes y enfermedades serias no ocurrirán. F M D

49. Me da terror ir a un sitio nuevo o encontrar un grupo nuevo de gente. F M D

50. Creo que es horrible encontrar la posibilidad de morirme. F M D

Glossary

abandono del hogar: Abandonment of the home—a Mexican law that penalizes a woman for leaving her home, even if domestic violence occurs.

abrazo: Embrace or hug.

aguantar: To endure; put up with.

los biles: "Pochismo" (adoption of English words into Spanish) for bills that have to be paid each month.

los blanquillos: Euphemism for eggs, "little white ones," to avoid a slang reference to testicles.

botanica: Store in a Spanish-speaking neighborhood where a variety of healing plants and ritual healing objects are sold.

brujeria: Witchcraft; belief in hexes and magical techniques to achieve goals.

carga emocional: Stress; literally "emotional heaviness."

casa chica: A second home where a man maintains a mistress and often children in addition to his home with a wife or common-law spouse.

cholo, chola: Derogatory term for gang member, with connotations of violence.

cochinada: Piglike; abominable.

confianza: Trust or confidence in a therapeutic relationship as well as with others.

consentido: Children who are badly spoiled, lacking any rules or discipline in the home.

cuentas: Bills or accounts to be paid.

Curanderismo: Folk medical treatment found throughout Latin America.

curandero: Traditional folk healer, becoming more common in some parts of the United States, using plants and other medicines and techniques.

daño: Physical harm due to bewitchment by an evildoer.

desechable: Throwaway, as in a useless child who does not help you.

desesperacíon: Desperation; reported by depressed clients.

dichos: Proverbs, sayings.

empacho: Folk illness affecting children.

envidia: Envy of others.

espiritista: Religious activity and belief that the living can contact the spirits of the dead.

guiso: Stew; meal.

haciendado: A hacienda or plantation owner.

huevo: Egg.

indio: Indian appearance; used disrespectfully.

juramento: Vow before the Virgin, generally by men who plan to give up drinking alcohol.

loco: Crazy, insane.

mal aire: Evil air, believed to cause illness to both adults and children.

marianismo: A cult of the Virgin Mary, generally resulting in a type of martyrdom for females.

marido: Latin American term for common-law spouse, although sometimes used for legal spouse.

muelle: Dock or slip for a boat.

mujer: Woman, wife.

los nervios: Nerves; used to describe a feeling of deep depression.

parece mentira: A paradox; it may appear to be a lie, but it is not.

personalismo: A relationship of trust when two individuals value the worth of each other; not dependent upon material wealth.

piropo: Flirtatious compliment, at times negative, made by men to women.

rancho: Ranch, small farm or hamlet.

remedio casero: Home remedy for illness.

respeto: Important value in Latino cultures of respect, regard, and consideration for others.

simpático: Well-liked individual who is sympathetic to the needs and desires of others.

susto: Fright or scare.

el truco: "Pocho" term for a truck instead of the Spanish word *camion.*

usted (Vd.): Polite form of address, meaning "you."

vicio: Vice, such as drinking, smoking, etc.

vidente: Seer or prophet.

vocero, vocera: Spokesperson.

voluntad: Willpower.

References

Alberti, Robert and Michael Emmons (1995). *Your perfect right: A guide to assertive living* (Seventh edition). Atascadero, CA: Impact Publishers.

Araujo, Jess (1998). *La ley y sus derechos.* Santa Ana, CA.

Atkinson, D.R. (1983). Ethnic similarity in counseling psychology: A review of research. *Counseling Psychologist,* 11(4):79-92.

Balon, R., V.K. Yeragani, R. Pohl, and C. Ramesh (1993). Sexual dysfunction during antidepressant treatment. *Journal of Clinical Psychiatry,* 54:209-212.

Barkley, Russell and Christine M. Benton (1997). *Niños desafiantes: Materiales de evaluacion y folletos para los padres.* Trans. José Banermeister. New York: Guilford Press.

Beck, A.T., A.J. Rush, B.F. Shaw, and G. Emery (1979). *Cognitive therapy of depression.* New York: Guilford Press.

Bem, Sandra L. (1981). Gender schema theory: A cognitive account of sex typing. *Psychological Review,* 88(3):354-364.

Berlin, Richard, Mary E. Olson, Carlos Cano, and Susan Engel (1991). Metaphor and psychotherapy. *American Journal of Psychotherapy,* 45(3):359-367.

Berry, J.W. (1993). Ethnic identity in plural societies. In M.E. Bernal and G.P. Knight (Eds.), *Ethnic identity formation and transformation among Hispanics and other minorities* (pp. 124-137). Albany, NY: SUNY Press.

Bibeau, Gilles (1997). Cultural psychiatry in a creolizing world: Questions for a new research agenda. *Transcultural Psychiatry,* 34(1):90-141.

Brody, C.M. (1987). The white therapist and female minority clients: Gender and cultural issues. *Psychotherapy,* 24(1):108-113.

Caetano, R. (1989). Drinking patterns and alcohol problems in a national sample of U.S. Hispanics. In D. Spengler (Ed.). *Alcohol use among U.S. ethnic minorities* (pp. 99-123). National Institute on Alcohol Abuse and Alcoholism, Research Monograph number 18. DHHS Public. number (ADM) 89-1435. Washington, DC: U.S. Government Printing Office.

Campbell, Joseph (1973). *Myths to live by.* London: Souvenir Press.

Canino, Gloria (1982). The Hispanic woman: Sociocultural influences on diagnosis and treatment. In R. Becerra, (Ed.), *Mental health and Hispanic Americans* (pp. 86-103). New York: Grune & Stratton.

Casas, J. Manuel, R. Burl Wagenheim, Robert Banchero, and Juan Mendoze-Romero (1994). Hispanic masculinity: Myth or psychological schema meriting clinical consideration? In Lillian Comas-Diaz and Beverly Greene (Eds.), *Women of color: Integrating ethnic and gender identities in psychotherapy* (pp. 407-418). New York: Guilford Press.

Castenada, Xochitl, Victor Ortiz, Allen Betania, Cecilia Gracia, and Mauricio Hernandez-Avila (1996). Sex masks: The double life of female commercial sex workers in Mexico City. *Culture, Medicine, and Psychiatry,* 20(2):229-247.

Cervantes, R.C., M.J. Gilbert, V.N. Slagado de Snyder, and A.M. Padilla (1990). Psychosocial and cognitive correlates of alcohol use in younger adult immigrants and U.S. born Hispanics. *International Journal of the Addictions,* 25 (5-6):689-710.

Cole, Michael (1996). *Cultural psychology.* Cambridge, MA: Harvard University Press.

Comas-Diaz, Lillian (1992). The future of psychotherapy with ethnic minorities. *Psychotherapy,* 29(1):88-165.

Comas-Diaz, Lillian and Beverly Greene (1994). Overview: Gender and ethnicity in the healing process. In Lillian Comas-Diaz and Beverly Greene (Eds.), *Women of color: Integrating ethnic and gender identities in psychotherapy* (pp. 3-35). New York: Guilford Press.

Comas-Diaz, Lillian and E.E.H. Griffith (Eds.) (1988). *Clinical guidelines in cross-cultural mental health.* New York: Wiley.

Combs, Gene and Jill Freedman (1990). *Symbol, story, and ceremony: Using metaphor in individual and family therapy.* New York: W.W. Norton.

Cushman, Phillip (1990). Why the self is empty: Toward a historically situated psychology. *American Psychologist,* 45(4):599-611.

de Rios, Marlene Dobkin (1972). *Visionary vine: Psychedelic healing in the Peruvian Amazon.* San Francisco: Chandler Publishing Company.

de Rios, Marlene Dobkin (1984a). *Hallucinogens: Cross-cultural perspective.* Albuquerque, NM: University of New Mexico Press.

de Rios, Marlene Dobkin (1984b). The *vidente* phenomenon in third world traditional healing: An Amazonian example. *Medical Anthropology,* 8(1):60-70.

de Rios, Marlene Dobkin (1985). Saladera: A culture-bound misfortune syndrome in the Peruvian Amazon. In Ronald C. Simons and Charles C. Hughes (Eds.), *The culture-bound syndromes: Folk illness of psychiatric and anthropological interest* (pp. 279-288). Dordrecht: Reidel Publishing Company.

de Rios, Marlene Dobkin (1992). *Amazon healer: The life and times of an urban shaman.* Dorset, England: Prism Press.

de Rios, Marlene Dobkin (1997). Magical realism: A cultural intervention for traumatized Hispanic children. *Cultural diversity and Mental Health,* 3(3):159-170.

de Rios, Marlene Dobkin and Bruce Achauer (1990). Pain relief for Hispanic burn patients using cultural metaphors. *Plastic and Reconstructive Surgery,* 17(1): 54-59.

de Rios, Marlene Dobkin and Daniel Feldman (1976). An anthropological approach to the study of minority drinking problems. Newsletter, California Society for the Treatment of Alcoholism and Drug Dependencies, 3(3):5-6.

de Rios, Marlene Dobkin and Daniel Feldman (1977). Southern California Mexican American drinking patterns: Some preliminary observations. *Journal of Psychoactive Drugs*, 9(2):151-158.

de Rios, Marlene Dobkin and Joyce Friedman (1987). Hypnotherapy with Hispanic burn patients. *International Journal of Clinical and Experimental Hypnosis*, 35 (2):87-94.

de Rios, Marlene Dobkin and Joyce Friedman (1990). Pain control and systematic desensitization inductions in Spanish for symptoms of post-traumatic stress disorder. In D. Corydon Hammond (Ed.), *Handbook of hypnotic suggestions and metaphors* (pp. 453-456). New York: W.W. Norton. American Society of Clinical Hypnosis.

de Rios, Marlene Dobkin, Andrei Novac, and Bruce H. Achauer (1997). Sexual dysfunction and the patient with burns. *Journal of Burn Care and Rehabilitation*, 18(1):37-42.

de Rios, Marlene Dobkin and Michael Winkelman (1989) (Eds.), Special theme issue, "Trance and shamanism." *Journal of Psychoactive Drugs*, 21(1).

Dinkmeyer, Don Sr., Gary D. McKay, and Don Dinkmeyer Jr. (1997). *The parents' handbook: Systematic training for effective parenting*. Circle Pines, MN: American Guidance Service, Inc.

Dolan, Yvonne M. (1986). Metaphors for motivation and intervention. In Steve de Shazer and John Kral (Eds.), *Indirect approaches in therapy* (pp. 225-231). Rockville, MD: Aspen Publications.

Fabrega, Horacio (1995). Hispanic mental health research: A case for cultural psychiatry. In Amado Padilla (Ed.), *Hispanic psychology* (pp. 107-130). Thousand Oaks, CA: Sage Publishing.

Falicov, Celia Taes (1998). *Latino families in therapy: A guide to multicultural practice*. New York: Guilford Press.

Favazza, Armando (1980). Culture change and mental health. *Journal of Operational Psychiatry*, 11(1):101-119.

Fodor, I.G. (1988). Cognitive behavior therapy: Evaluation of theory and practice for addressing women's issues. In M.A. Dutton-Douglas and L.E. Walker (Eds.), *Feminist psychotherapies: Integration of therapeutic and feminist systems* (pp. 347-359). Norwood, NJ: Ablex Publishing.

Freedman, Jill and Gene Combs (1996). *Narrative therapy: The social construction of preferred realities*. New York: W.W. Norton and Company.

Freud, Sigmund [1900](1953). The interpretation of dreams. In James Strachey (Ed.), *The standard edition of the complete works of Sigmund Freud*, Volumes 4 and 5. London: Hogarth Press.

Gardner, John (1971). *Therapeutic communication with children: The mutual storytelling technique*. New York: Jason Aronson.

Gilmore, M. and D. Gilmore (1990). Machismo: A psychodynamic approach (Spain). *Journal of Psychological Anthropology*. 2:281-299.

Ginorio, A. and J. Reno (1986). Violence in the lives of Latina women. In M.C. Burns (Ed.), *The speaking profits vs. violence in the lives of women of color* (pp. 89-93). Seattle, WA: Center for the Prevention of Sexual and Domestic Violence.

Gonzalez, Roberto Cortez, Joan L. Biever, and Glen T. Gardner (1973). *The multicultural perspective in therapy: A social constructionist approach.* Presented at 10th Annual Teachers College Winter Roundtable on Crosscultural Counseling and Psychotherapy. Columbia, NY, February.

Grove, David (1989). *Resolving traumatic memories: Metaphors and symbols in psychotherapy.* New York: Irvington Publishers.

Harris, Mary G. (1987). Cholas—Mexican-American gang girls. Bloomsburg University Department of Curriculum and Foundation, Bloomsburg, PA. Unpublished manuscript.

Helman, Cecil (1994). *Culture, health, and illness* (Third edition). London: Butterworth Heineman.

Helzer, John E. and Glorisa J. Canino (Eds.) (1992). *Alcoholism in North America, Europe, and Asia.* New York: Oxford University Press.

Hilgard, Ernest R. and Josephine R. Hilgard (1983). *Hypnosis in the relief of pain* (Revised edition). Los Altos, CA: William Kaufmann, Inc.

Howard, George S. (1991). Culture tales: A narrative approach to thinking, cross-cultural psychology, and psychotherapy. *American Psychologist,* 46(3):187-197.

Jenkins, J.H. and Marvin Karno (1992). The meaning of expressed emotion: Theoretical issues raised by cross-cultural research. *American Journal of Psychiatry,* 149:9-21.

Kanuha, Valli (1994). Women of color in battering relationships. In Lillian Comas-Diaz and Beverly Greene (Eds.), *Women of color* (pp. 455-463). New York: Guilford Press.

Karno, Marvin and Robert B. Edgerton (1969). Perceptions of mental illness in a Mexican-American community. *Archives of General Psychiatry,* 20(4):233-238.

Kleinman, Arthur (1980). *Patients and healers in the context of culture.* Berkeley, CA: University of California Press.

Knight, Helen (1997). U.S. immigration level at highest peak since 1930s. *Los Angeles Times,* April 9, p. A17.

Kopp, Richard R. (1995). *Metaphor therapy: Using client-generated metaphors in psychotherapy.* New York: Tavistock.

Lankton, Carol H. and Stephen R. Lankton (1989). *Tales of enchantment.* New York: Brunner/Mazel.

Lewis, Sandra Y. (1994). Cognitive-behavioral therapy. In Amado Padilla (Ed.), *Hispanic psychology* (pp. 372-385). Newbury Park, CA: Sage Focus Editions.

Lin, Keh-Min, Russell E. Poland, and Dora Anderson (1995). Psychopharmacology, ethnicity, and culture. *Transcultural Psychiatric Research Review,* 32(1):3-40.

Mauss, Marcel [1885](1973). *The gift: Forms and functions of exchange in archaic society.* London: Cohen and West.

Mayers, Raymond Sanchez (1989). The use of folk medicine by elderly Mexican-American women. *Journal of Drug Issues*, 19(2):283-295.

McCarney, Stephen B. (1994). *Formulario de evaluación en version doméstica*. Columbia, MO: Hawthorne Educational Services, Inc.

McCarney, Stephen and Angela Marie Bauer (1994). *A parent's guide to children with attention deficit and hyperactivity disroder*. Columbia, MO: Hawthorne Educational Services.

McGrath, E., G.P. Keita, B.R. Strickland, and N.F. Russo (1990). *Women and depression: Risk factors and treatment issues*. Final Report, American Psychological Association. National Task Force on Women and Depression. Washington, DC: American Psychological Association.

McKenna, Matthew, Eugene McCray, and Ida Onorato (1995). The epidemiology of tuberculosis among foreign-born persons in the U.S., 1986-1993. *New England Journal of Medicine*, 332(16):1071-1077.

Mills, Joyce and Richard J. Crowley (1986). *Therapeutic metaphors for children and the child within*. New York: Brunner/Mazel.

Moerman, Daniel E. (1979). Anthropology of symbolic healing. *Current Anthropology*, 20(1):59-80.

Moscicki, E., B. Locke, D. Rae, and J. Boyd (1989). Depressive symptoms among Mexican Americans. *American Journal of Epidemiology*, 130(3):348-360.

Murphy, H.B.M. (1969). Ethnic variations in drug responses. *Transcultural Psychiatric Research Review*, 6(1):6-23.

National Center for Health Statistics (1987). Health care coverage by age, sex, race and family income. Advance Data, Number 139, September 18, 1987. Washington, DC: U.S. Government Printing Office.

Padilla, Amado M. (Ed.) (1994). *Hispanic psychology: Critical issues in theory and research*. Newbury Park, CA: Sage Focus Editions.

Paz, Octavio (1980). *Labyrinth of solitude: Life and thought in Mexico*. New York: Evergreen Books.

Pederson, P. (1991). Multiculturalism as a generic approach to counseling. *Journal of Counseling and Development*, 70:6-12.

Piaget, Jean (1969). *The psychology of the child*. Cambridge, MA: Basic Books.

Pleck, Joseph (1981). *The myth of masculinity*. Cambridge, MA: MIT Press.

Polcin, Douglas (1995). Integrating 12-step approaches into therapy with substance abusers: An examination of controversial issues. *California Therapist*, 7(1):83-97.

Polcin, Douglas L. (1997). Combining cognitive behavioral and 12-step approaches in the treatment of alcohol dependence. *California Therapist*, 9(2):47-51.

Polster, Ervin and Miriam Polster (1973). *Gestalt therapy integrated*. New York: Brunner/Mazel.

Quintana, Stephen (1995). Acculturative stress: Latino immigrants and the counseling profession. *Counseling Psychologist*, 23(1):68-73.

Rivera, George Jr. (1990). AIDS and Mexican folk medicine. *Social Science Research*, 75(1):3-7.

Rossi, Ernest (1986). *The psychobiology of mind-body healing.* New York: W.W. Norton.

Rouse, Beatrice, James H. Carter, and Sylvia Rodriquez-Andrew (1995). Race, ethnicity, and other sociocultural influences on alcoholism treatment for women. In Marc Galanter (Ed.), *Recent developments in alcoholism* (pp. 293-298). New York: Plenum Press.

Ruiz, Pedro (1995). Assessing, diagnosing, and treating culturally diverse individuals: A Hispanic perspective. *Psychiatric Quarterly,* 66(4):329-341.

Schoef, Caroline (1995). Cultural stigma and self-esteem of Mexican mentally retarded children in two cities. Unpublished MA thesis. California State University, Fullerton.

Schumaker, John F. (1995). *The corruption of reality: A unified theory of religion, hypnosis, and psychopathology.* Amherst, NY: Prometheus Books.

Seale, J.P., J.F. Williams, and N. Amodei (1992). Alcoholism prevalence and utilization of medical services by Mexican Americans. *Journal of Family Practice,* 35(2):169-174.

Seligman, Martin P. (1975). *Helplessness: On depression, development, and death.* San Francisco: Freeman Publishers.

Sheik, Aneesh (Ed.) (1984). *Imagination and healing.* Farmingdale, NY: Baywood Publishing Company.

Short, Patrick, Gloria Camino, Hector Bird, Maritza Rubio-Stipec, Milagros Bravo, and M. Audrey Buman (1994). Mental health status among Puerto Ricans, Mexican Americans, and non-Hispanic whites. *American Journal of Community Psychology,* 20(6):729-752.

Shweder, Richard A. and Edmund J. Bourne (1982). Does the concept of the person vary cross-culturally? In A.J. Marsella and G.M. White (Eds.), *Cultural conceptions of mental health and therapy* (pp. 97-137). Chicago: University of Chicago Press.

Shweder, Richard and L. LeVine (Eds.) (1984). *Culture theory: Essays in mind, theory, and emotion.* Cambridge, England: Cambridge University Press.

Siegelman, Ellen Y. (1990). *Metaphor and meaning in psychotherapy.* New York: Guilford Press.

Simoni, Jane M. and Leonor Perez (1995). Latinos and mutual support groups: A case for considering culture. *American Journal of Orthopsychiatry,* 65(3):440-445.

Singer, Helen Kaplan (1974). *The new sex therapy.* New York: Brunner/Mazel.

Smart, Jule and David W. Smart (1995). Acculturative stress: The experience of the Hispanic immigrant. *Counseling Psychologist,* 23(1):25-42.

Southern California Association of Governments (1984). *Projections of population demographics in the coming 50 years.* Unpublished report.

Stigler, James W., Richard A. Shweder, and Gilbert Herdt (Eds.) (1990). *Cultural psychology: Essays on comparative human development.* Cambridge, England: Cambridge University Press.

Suarez-Orozco, M. and A. Dundes (1984). The *piropo* and the dual image of women in the Spanish-speaking world. *Journal of Latin American Lore,* 10(1):111-133.

Sue, Deward W. (1992). The challenge of multiculturalism: The road less traveled. *American Counselor,* 1(1):6-10, 12-14.

Sullivan, Karen Riddle (1992). A comparison of Hispanic American and Anglo-American battered women. Unpublished MA thesis, California State University, Fullerton.

Szapocznik, José and William M. Kurtines (1993). Family psychology and cultural diversity: Opportunities for theory, research, and application. *American Psychologist,* 48(4):400-407.

Thorne-Finch, R. (1992). *Ending the silence: The origins and treatment of male violence against women.* Toronto: University of Toronto Press.

Torrey, E. Fuller (1972). *The mind game: Witchdoctors and psychiatrists.* New York: Emerson Hall.

Triandis, H.C., G. Marin, J. Lisansky, and H. Betancourt (1984). *Simpatia* as a cultural script of Hispanics. *Journal of Personality and Social Psychology,* 47(4):1363-1375.

U.S. Bureau of the Census (1991). Resident population distribution for the U.S. region and state by race and Hispanic origin. 1990. Census Bureau Press Release number CB 91-100. Washington, DC: U.S. Government Printing Office.

U.S. Department of Justice (1992). Immigration reform and control act. Report on the legalized alien population. Immigration and Naturalization Service. Washington, DC: U.S. Government Printing Office.

Vargas, Luis A. and Joan K. Koss-Chioino (Eds.) (1992). *Working with culture: Psychotherapeutic interventions with ethnic minority children and adolescents.* San Francisco: Jossey-Bass.

Vasquez, Carmen and Rafael A. Javier (1991). The problem with interpreters: Communicating with Spanish-speaking patients. *Hospital and Community Psychiatry,* 42(2):163-165.

Vasquez, Melba (1994). Latinas. In Lillian Comas-Diaz and Beverly Greene (Eds.), *Women of color* (pp. 78-92). New York: Guilford Press.

Vega, W.A., B. Kolody, and R. Valle (1987). Migration and mental health: An empirical test of depression risk factors among Mexican American women. *International Migration Review,* 21(4):512-529.

Vega, W.A., B. Kolody, R. Valle, and J. Weir (1991). Social networks, social support, and their relationship to depression among immigrant Mexican women. *Human Organization,* 50(3):154-162.

Verdonk, A. (1979). Migration and mental illness. *International Journal of Social Psychiatry,* 25:295-305.

Walsh, Roger (1989). The shamanic journey: Experiences, origins, and analogues. *ReVision,* 12(2):25-32.

Weisinger, Hendrie (1985). *Dr. Weisinger's anger work-out book.* New York: Quill Press.

Weissman, Alicia M. (1994). Preventive health care and screening of Latin American immigrants in the U.S. *Journal of the American Board of Family Practice,* 7(4):310-323.

Williams, J.A. (1973). Voluntary associations and minority status: A comparative analysis of Anglo, Black and Mexican Americans. *American Sociological Review*, 38(3):637-647.

Winkelman, Michael (1989). Cross-cultural study of shamanistic healers. *Journal of Psychoactive Drugs*, 21(1):17-24.

Winkelman, Michael (1993). *Ethnic relations in the U.S.: A sociohistorical cultural systems approach.* St. Paul, MN: West Publishing Company.

Wolfe, J.L. and I.G. Fodor (1975). A cognitive/behavioral approach to modifying assertive behavior in women. *Counseling Psychologist*, 54(4):5-59.

World Health Organization (1986). Dose effects of antidepressant medication in different populations. *Journal of Affective Disorders*, (Supp. 2), 1-67.

Zuniga, Maria (1991). Dichos as metaphorical tools for resistant Latino clients. *Psychotherapy*, 28(3):480-483.

Index

Page numbers followed by the letter "i" indicate illustrations; those followed by the letter "t" indicate tables.

T - #0546 - 101024 - C0 - 212/152/11 - PB - 9780789010902 - Gloss Lamination